The Person in Narrative Therapy

Palgrave Studies in the Theory and History of Psychology

Palgrave Studies in the *Theory and History of Psychology* publishes scholarly books that use historical and theoretical methods to critically examine the historical development and contemporary status of psychological concepts, methods, research, theories, and interventions. The books in the series are characterised by an emphasis on the concrete particulars of psychologists' scientific and professional practices, together with a critical examination of the assumptions that attend their use. These examinations are anchored in clear, accessible descriptions of what psychologists do and believe about their activities. All the books in the series share the general goal of advancing the scientific and professional practices of psychology and psychologists, even as they offer probing and detailed questioning and critical reconstructions of these practices.

Titles include:

Michael Guilfoyle
THE PERSON IN NARRATIVE THERAPY
A Post-structural, Foucauldian Account

Palgrave Studies in the Theory and History of Psychology
Series Standing Order ISBN 978–1–137–34443–4 Hardback
(*outside North America only*)

You can receive future titles in this series as they are published by placing a standing order. Please contact your bookseller or, in case of difficulty, write to us at the address below with your name and address, the title of the series and the ISBN quoted above.

Customer Services Department, Macmillan Distribution Ltd, Houndmills, Basingstoke, Hampshire RG21 6XS, England

The Person in Narrative Therapy

A Post-structural, Foucauldian Account

Michael Guilfoyle
Psychology Department, Rhodes University, South Africa

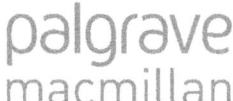

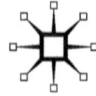
First published 2014 by
PALGRAVE MACMILLAN

Palgrave Macmillan in the UK is an imprint of Macmillan Publishers Limited, registered in England, company number 785998, of Houndmills, Basingstoke, Hampshire RG21 6XS.

Palgrave Macmillan in the US is a division of St Martin's Press LLC, 175 Fifth Avenue, New York, NY 10010.

Palgrave Macmillan is the global academic imprint of the above companies and has companies and representatives throughout the world.

Palgrave® and Macmillan® are registered trademarks in the United States, the United Kingdom, Europe and other countries.

ISBN 978–1–137–38054–8

This book is printed on paper suitable for recycling and made from fully managed and sustained forest sources. Logging, pulping and manufacturing processes are expected to conform to the environmental regulations of the country of origin.

A catalogue record for this book is available from the British Library.

A catalog record for this book is available from the Library of Congress.

Contents

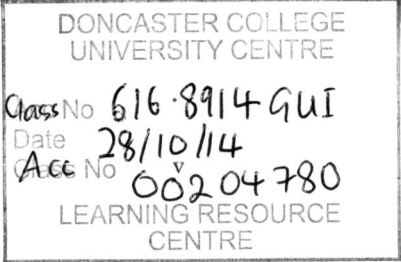

Acknowledgements

To my wife and best friend, Trudy Meehan, one of the smartest people I know. Thank you for not agreeing with me on so many occasions, for pushing me to rethink and to be clearer, and for always believing that I had something important to say. I am inspired by your ability to model resistance and agency in the face of a world that's not always kind, and not always fair. For what it's worth, this is for you.

I am also very grateful to Ed, Sydney, and Blue, for loving me, and for nudging me away from the computer every now and then. My mom and dad, two of the most ethical human beings I know, as well as Kelly, Richard, Andrew, and Shanna.

Thank you to my colleagues all around the world. There are three groups to whom I am particularly grateful for giving me space to share my narrative practice experiences, and for sharing their own experiences with me in turn. My peer supervision group in Dublin, Ireland: Paul Kelly, Paidraic Gibson, and Tony Horgan. The Dublin narrative therapy group: Therese Hegarty, Paul Heslin, Marie Keenen, Ann Campbell, Nora Sweetman, Trish Tyrrell, Margaruete Kirwan, Keith Oulton, and all those others I met along the way. And then the Grahamstown Narrative Therapy Network: Jan Knoetze, Lisl Foss, Ilse Appelt, Kim Barker, Linda Schwartz, Trudy Meehan, Zimbini Ogle, Lucia Oosthuysen, and Lindsay Smaill. Emerging from that group, Lisl and I had many stimulating conversations about the strengths and limitations of narrative practice. Thank you, Lisl, for standing alongside me as I jumped from my safe perch. You helped me to teach, practise, and in some ways even live more openly and honestly. I am so pleased to have friends in you, Richard, and Torey, who nurture us with meals and conversation when we most need it.

Special mention must go to Judy Rankin, Ruby Patel, and Floss Mitchell, for always treating me like a human being.

I have learned much from the students with whom I have worked over the years, and who stretched me across some kind of zone of proximal development, at both Trinity College Dublin (Ireland) and Rhodes University (South Africa). I would like to make special mention of the 2012 M1 students of the Counselling Psychology Master's programme at Rhodes University: Kirsten Farquharson, Donna Mitchell, Thobeka

Msengana, Jeremy Ruiters, Lindsay Smaill, and Beverly Texeira. You pushed me to think through my ideas more clearly, and always to make them relevant to the people with whom we work. It is with you, during our Tuesday conversations, that many of these ideas began to come to life.

I tip my hat to Tim Barry, Kevin Durrheim, Graham Lindegger, Doug Wassenaar, Anthony Pillay, David Ingleby, and Len Holdstock: my intellectual stimulants. We haven't always kept in touch, but over the years you have inspired me, believed in me, and pushed my thinking to places I never thought it could go.

I am grateful to Rhodes University, for giving me the time and space needed to complete this book, to series editor Jack Martin, for offering very useful suggestions regarding what I needed to clarify, and to Nicola Jones, editor, for guiding me through the publishing process with kindness, wisdom, and patience.

And then, to the people with whom I have worked over the last 24 years. None of the stories I tell are about you, and yet your mark on my thinking pervades the book. Your stories of pain, trauma, misery, hope, celebration, connection, humility, courage, determination, and resolve have touched my life in ways I cannot easily put into words. You have shown me a million ways in which ethics, values, and commitments can be brought to life. In my eyes you have contributed to an enrichment of the world, and inspired not only my thought but also my ways of being. Thank you for making therapy such a wonderful lifetime journey for me.

This work is based upon research supported by the National Research Foundation (NRF, South Africa). Any opinions, findings, and conclusions or recommendations expressed in this material are those of the author, and therefore the NRF does not accept any liability in regard thereto.

Introduction

On the face of it, this is a book about theory. But it is also a book about practice. My aim is to use theory to show that narrative practice can embrace a range of voices, styles, and ethics. This grand ambition flows from my initial and far more personal goal to situate myself as a practitioner; not as a facsimiled, degraded version of Michael White – genius though he undoubtedly was – but as a post-structurally oriented narrative practitioner with my own unique voice, style, ethos, and even ethics. This book is part of my attempt to find myself in this way.

My frustration at my own difficulties in working as a narrative therapist has its own particular history. I trained as a clinical psychologist in the late 1980s, during which time I was exposed to the exciting ideas of such figures as Minuchin, Whitaker, Bateson, Erickson, and the members of the Milan School. Then, in the early 1990s, following a trajectory that is probably shared by many others in the narrative therapy world, I – in partnership with and inspired by my gifted friend, Tim Barry – encountered social constructionist and narrative ideas. I excitedly read the works of such authors as Tom Andersen, Kenneth Gergen, Sheila McNamee, Lynn Hoffman, and, of course, Michael White and David Epston. This led me to seek out further training in narrative therapy and in the supervision of narrative practices, as I simultaneously tried in different settings to teach these ideas to students as well as to put them into practice.

But I always experienced a sense of unease, which I could only really begin to articulate in the mid-2000s: after over a decade of considering myself a narrative therapist, I still couldn't quite do it the way that White or Epston seemed to. A colleague of mine told me that he went into narrative therapy training because he 'wanted to be able to do what Michael and David did'. But I could never do what they did. My clients just weren't responding the right way! Was I doing it wrong? While I felt that my work was reasonably effective, more often than not it seemed that client change was linked with something other than my narrative 'moves'; the nature of the relationship, for example, seemed far more influential.

What confused the matter further was the insistence of narrative therapy figures – colleagues, workshop facilitators, journal editors, and reviewers – that narrative therapy was not about 'technique', but a way of thinking, and a way of being with a client. Hearing such characterizations, I concluded that I must indeed be doing it wrong, thinking about it incorrectly, or even 'being' wrong. The trouble was not that I disagreed with the intentions of these characterizations. Quite the reverse, in fact: I agreed that a focus on 'technique' could be sterile, and I took the relationship with the client very seriously indeed. And, yet, I still couldn't get the hang of certain practices, especially 'externalizing the problem', which I found trickiest of all. I had to tell myself – and my students – 'externalizing is not a technique, but a way of thinking'. But such assertions weren't terribly convincing, and I felt I was forcing myself (and my students) to accept a principle upon which so many insisted, but which seemed incongruent with my own experience. My experience was telling me that narrative therapy was an awful lot about technique.

Consider, for example, that probably the most currently influential narrative therapy text (White's [2007] *Maps of Narrative Practice*) is structured around – and provides a structure for – seven 'maps' for hosting and guiding conversations. Is there really any significant difference between 'maps' and 'techniques'? White says there is, but I'm not so sure. In each case one has pre-constructed procedures or steps to follow that move the client from point A to B. It is true that many of these maps have proven useful in my own practice. But occasionally I feel, as I move into one or other conversational map, that I am stepping onto a pathway that has already been laid out. It is not mine, nor is it my client's: it is, to be frank, Michael White's. It is indeed a beautiful, exciting, and productive pathway. But I am always aware that someone else has already levelled the ground and cleared away the bushes and thorns; even put their own signposts on it. This takes away just a fraction of the sheen of the pathway, at least for me. This matters when, sometimes, I get knocked out of the immediacy of my relationship with the client, as I become aware of what lurks around the next corner: a question about hopes and dreams, perhaps? What will she say when we get to the part where we discuss values and commitments? And then sometimes it feels as though the client is going along the 'mapped' pathway with me, but somewhat reluctantly. Worse, my questions around my sense of the client's reluctance seldom yield a productive conversation: 'No, no, it's fine! You're the expert!' says the person, reproducing all of the hierarchical ideas I have spent much of my career trying to unsettle. I have a sense that the client allows us to follow this pathway as a courtesy to me, or as a form of deference to my own supposed wisdom. And this is a difficult deference to overcome.

I should emphasize that this has been my personal experience, and I do not assume that it is shared by others. In fact, many practitioners have told me of the ease with which they engage in re-authoring or re-membering practices with others, of the sense of 'flow' that sometimes accompanies those dialogues, and of their feeling of personal congruence when working as narrative therapists. I have envied these people, and for many years tortured myself with the question: 'Why can't I do it?'

I finally decided to reject the view that I am simply incompetent, not sufficiently trained, not smart enough, or in the wrong profession. I also learned over time that the solution, for me, does not lie in identifying with another approach (despite my flirtations with relational psychoanalysis, and interpersonal and existential psychotherapies). Indeed, a big part of my difficulty was that I was, and remain, committed to the theoretical and philosophical foundations of narrative practice; something I will discuss in some depth in this book. So what could I do about my powerful sense of philosophical and epistemological alignment, in the context of my experience in practice of trying to squeeze myself into an outfit that seems to have been designed for someone else?

The turning point for me came when I realized I was asking the wrong questions. For many years I was trying to figure out: 'What would a good narrative therapist do here?'; 'Why are my clients not following the logic of my questions?'; 'How can I improve my externalizing practices?'; 'How should I follow this conversational map?' These are questions about 'technique'. However, my attempts to answer them left me feeling stifled rather than liberated as a practitioner, and I began to doubt my own competence. So, I changed tack, and began trying to tackle a very different kind of question: not 'What should I do?', but 'Who are *you*? What have you been made into? How would you like to live?' This led to other questions: 'Who is the person in narrative therapy? What sort of world does she or he occupy, and what impact does this have on him or her?' I began to de-privilege the question of how to 'do' good narrative therapy, and became more curious about how I should think about the person sitting in front of me, and about how she or he is situated in relation to the social world, with its multiple power dynamics and social pressures. And then, given these understandings, I can face the task of trying to engage usefully with him or her.

This orientation to the person as one who lives in the context of a social universe understood in a particular (more or less Foucauldian) way – an orientation, we might say, to the person-in-power – seemed to me a potentially solid platform from which to conduct my own work as a therapist. This book is an attempt to articulate some of my efforts to address that question. In the process, I feel I have become able to approach narrative work in a different way: by trying to understand the dynamics of the person-in-power, rather than by tracing Michael White's (2007) 'maps', or by modelling on his, or David Epston's, brilliant therapeutic interventions.

This shift in my overall, orienting question has opened up my experience of narrative work significantly, at both a theoretical and a practical level.

At the level of theory, the work of Michel Foucault, and that of some of his contemporaries and predecessors, such as Nietzsche, Deleuze, Veyne, and Klossowski, took on new significance for me. I decided to begin looking at the question of the person from a philosophical perspective. I was interested to see that there are authors who have written specifically on the question of the Foucauldian human being, or the Foucauldian subject. This in turn led me to the work of Pierre Klossowski, whose *Nietzsche and the Vicious Circle* was described by Foucault as the best philosophy text he had read, and Gilles Deleuze, whose text *Nietzsche and Philosophy* has been described as a key moment in the ushering in of post-structural thought. I also started reading Nietzsche – Foucault having always been a Nietzschean at heart (Veyne, 2010) – and began to make a different kind of sense of where Foucault was coming from. These authors offered some interesting clues about how to think about the person within a Nietzschean, post-structural context; clues that had not been taken up to any great extent in the narrative therapy literature, despite the insistence by White, Epston, and others that narrative therapy is a form of post-structural inquiry. So I became intrigued with the question of how post-structuralism might expand our thinking, as practitioners, about the person and his or her context.

These theoretical explorations led me to puzzle over the curious and creative tension between what has been described as the constituted subject on the one hand and the 'free', ethical subject on the other. That is, on the one hand, Foucauldian post-structuralism articulates the social forces that construct the person – expressed in extreme form in the idea of the individual as 'the product of power' (Foucault, 1983, p. xiv). Here, the person is considered a product of knowledge and power dynamics, an insight that inevitably shaped narrative therapists' sense of the person as constituted in stories (White, 1993), to such an extent that some hold that there is no a priori person behind the narrative (e.g., Madigan, 2010). This is in line with the Foucauldian sense of the person as constructed out of power and knowledge dynamics (both of which, incidentally, I see as incorporated in White's notion of 'narrative'). In its extreme form, this figure is portrayed as rather passive, docile, a puppet of the vicissitudes of power. It is no surprise then, that Foucault has been criticized for the impoverished vision of human agency implicit in much of his work.

Clearly, however, narrative therapy could not function with such a docile view of the human being, its alignment with Foucauldian post-structuralism notwithstanding. Agency has always been an essential part of narrative therapy's view of the person. But it has never been clear to me how this fits – if indeed it does – with the post-structuralism to which we have already committed ourselves. And so part of my intention here is to discuss various ways in which we might think of human agency, in ways that cohere with a Foucauldian and post-structural perspective. Some of my thinking about human agency involves an exploration of the 'human animal' that Foucault presupposed, but never really articulated, in his discussions of the constitutive forces of power/knowledge (O'Leary, 2002, p. 118). This is not an animal in the sense of one who acts out base instincts or drives, but an alive, dynamic being with its own capacities and abilities. And then, I turn to the personal agency implicit in what Foucault, in the last years of his life, referred to as the 'ethical subject': the figure who is able to engage reflexively and critically with the forces of social constitution; who can develop his or her own personal ethos, or style, together with a personalized sense of values and ethics.

Thus, the shift of my orienting question, away from issues of technique and towards a curiosity about what it means to be a person-in-power, has been associated with some interesting theoretical explorations. I will share some of these, but in doing so I will remain close to therapeutic problems and practices. This is, after all, a book about theory and practice and their mutual relevance. In particular, I have found these theoretical explorations useful in orienting to the person sitting across from me. They have helped me to sit more easily, and to feel that I don't have to always 'do' the clever bits of narrative therapy, or always be trying to transport the client to some new experiential territory of life. In any case, I feel that I am not always cognitively swift enough to facilitate this in the ways I have seen others do it. Instead, I can use as a platform for therapeutic work a vision of the person sitting across from me; a person who, in the first instance, has no choice but to exist in, and to make sense of him or herself with reference to a constraining but also productive social network of power and knowledge dynamics; as one who is, in other words, socially constituted. But this is also a person who possesses capacities, skills, knowledges, and the promise of a powerful value-base and set of personal commitments, all of which can help him or her deal more effectively with power and the ways in which it constructs him or her. I prefer to start at that point of understanding, rather than with my own seemingly limited skills in the prevailing narrative techniques or conversational maps.

I am not critical of the active, directed, and often creative work associated with White's narrative maps of practice, and I do admire, and am sometimes envious of, the elegant and seamless ways in which these were performed by White and others. My problem is only that they do not always sit easily with me, with my own timing and rhythm, or with my ways of being in relationship. And so I have tried to retrace some of our theoretical and philosophical steps in order to find narrative pathways that feel more accommodating of me. If I can sit reasonably comfortably, chances are my clients will benefit more from our work together.

In this book I articulate some of the theoretical and practical avenues through which I have been able to once again find myself on exciting therapeutic pathways with people. I have a better sense, now, not of the conversational map, or of how the path ahead looks or should look, but of the person alongside me. I can trust that he or she has the fundamental capacities to navigate and sometimes tame the rough terrains that lie ahead. *That* is the person I encounter.

The structure of the book is as follows: I begin with an orientation to the problem of personal agency versus constitution (Chapter 1), and proceed in Chapter 2 to discuss the power/knowledge complex which frames narrative therapeutic understandings of the world in which persons live out their lives. Chapter 3 examines the human subject that is produced in that kind of world. While the question of how persons resist the dictates of power on their identities and sense of self pervades the book, it is explored in some detail in the following two chapters. Chapter 4 explores White's and Foucault's beliefs that such resistance is a fundamentally social phenomenon, and I offer some critiques of their proposals. These critiques lead, in Chapter 5, to discussion of a human figure who is only implicit in Foucault's work, but without whom power/knowledge could not function. This is not the socially constituted being, but the embodied individual who precedes and escapes such constitution; an individual who is far more active, agentive, and resisting than Foucault's work typically suggests. Chapter 6 explores some implications of the preceding arguments for therapeutic practice. It proposes a narrative empathic approach, in which we hear the person not only as an agentive, active being, as is typical in narrative practice, but also as a constituted one. By empathizing with the person's sense of being trapped in a problem-saturated identity, we move closer to and witness his or her resisting capacities. Finally, Chapter 7 examines the dialogical development of these personal resistances, and proposes that narrative therapy helps thicken resistance into personal agency by orienting more to the ethics of the self than to the acquisition of self-knowledge. This assists persons in dealing more effectively with the power/knowledge systems that strive to manage their conduct and prescribe their identities.

1
The Problem: Constitution versus Agency

Who is the person in narrative therapy? And why do we not have a theory of the person in the way that our colleagues in psychoanalysis, in cognitive behavioural therapy, and in the humanistic or existential approaches have?

In *The Interpretation of Dreams*, Freud (1900) wrote: 'Everyone has wishes that he would prefer not to disclose to other people, and wishes that he will not even admit to himself' (p. 160). This statement captures what is often considered 'the ABC of psychoanalysis': a principle that unifies its approach to dreams, neuroses, psychoses, and everyday life (Borch-Jacobsen, 1988, p. 2). This is a view of the person as one who is constituted by the dynamic tensions between unconscious desires and wishes on the one side – those that cannot be admitted to oneself or to others – and the socialized, ordered, and integrating ego on the other. Out of this basic principle, it is possible to begin to formulate an understanding of the person. So fundamental is this principle that psychoanalytic textbooks typically outline some version of it, such that any undergraduate student could be expected to have an answer to the question: 'Who is the person in Freudian psychoanalysis?'

But the task is not so simple for the student or even the practitioner of narrative therapy. Why have we not developed an explicit formulation of the person? Our difficulty with this by-now standard practice in therapeutic theory stems from our understanding of knowledge and how it works. In this regard, we are indebted to the work of Michel Foucault, for whom knowledge (e.g., a theory of the person) is not an objective tool that represents reality in a neutral way, but a social product operating in the service of power dynamics. As such, knowledge should be seen not as a description of reality, but as a series of 'practices that systematically form the objects of which they speak' (Foucault, 1972, p. 49). Hence, for us, knowledge is not just a knowing, but a doing, which thereby ends up producing its articulations into social reality. A theory of the person is also a way of acting on the person.

Michael White (1993) echoes Foucault in his adoption of what he terms a 'constitutionalist perspective', which includes a rejection of the notion that the person can be known as an essential being; as one who is *this* or *that* in essence (p. 125). For White, this is a stance that

> refutes foundationalist assumptions of objectivity, essentialism, and representationalism. It proposes... that essentialist notions are paradoxical in that they provide descriptions that are specifying of life; that these notions obscure the operations of power. And the constitutionalist perspective proposes that the descriptions that we have of life are not representations or reflections of lives as lived, but are directly constitutive of life; that these descriptions... have real effects in the shaping of life.
>
> (1993, p. 125)

In a later work, White (2004) elaborates further on the dangers of claiming objective knowledge about the person. Any such knowledge, allowing the therapist to make the claim, 'This is who you *really* are', amounts in the end to a prescription, which presses the person to construct understandings of himself or herself in terms of that knowledge. White is concerned that the identification of a single organizing dynamic, principle, or force governing a person's life – such as we see in Freudian psychoanalysis – might promote a 'single-voiced' vision of the person, and limit his or her options for living (p. 135). Furthermore, in their stipulations of the 'true nature' of the person (p. 135), such knowledges promote norms which justify practices of exclusion, management, or control of those persons who seem to deviate from this natural standard of personhood.

Following this argument, then, we might suppose that Freud's psychoanalytic vision of the person is essentialist insofar as it alludes to some core dynamic that lies inherent in the person, that it misunderstands its own status as only a way of interpreting or representing the person, and that it thereby obscures from view the constitutive, prescriptive effects it has on persons' lives. Furthermore, its single-voiced nature – its reduction of human complexity and multiplicity to a few core principles – inevitably denigrates other possibilities for life, which may, for instance, be described in terms of denials, projections, somatizations, and so on, of the person's allegedly true unconscious wishes.

And lastly, the classical Freudian psychoanalytic view enables the construction of an entire social system of relations such that deviations from its prescriptions come to be socially devalued. For example, and as we shall see in the next chapter, psychoanalytic ways of knowing played a significant role in the pathologization of homosexuality, not just in the consulting room, but also in the broader culture. In principle, the same concerns could be expressed for any theoretical attempt to know the person.

It follows that the narrative practitioner should tread very carefully in this area. Neither Foucault nor White wishes to be in the business of personal and social control. And so our thought and our books tend to stay away from trying to answer too precisely this question: who is the person?

Nevertheless, I feel moved to ask it for two main reasons. First, it seems to me that we perform, even if we do not always articulate, certain understandings of the person in our practices. The intended influence and directionality of our practices – we engage with purpose – indicates our sense of knowing *something*, and this something is performed, despite our fears of its wide-ranging constitutive effects. What is this something that we know but seldom speak of? And second, I ask the question because, as I will argue throughout this work, the lack of a clear conceptualization of the person leaves the constitutionalist narrative approach with a significant limitation: it struggles to adequately account for the phenomena of personal agency and resistance. This means that it cannot properly explain one of the core conditions that must be met (i.e., an agentive, resisting human being) for its own practices to function.

And so I will attempt to work my way around the question, but, cognizant of White's warnings, I aim to do so without lapsing into an essentialist or normative position. In the process I will argue for a post-structural, multi-voiced account of the person which might usefully inform our narrative practices.

Foucault's human being and the problem of agency

If we are in some sense Foucauldian post-structuralists, and I think we are, we would do well to begin our journey by considering some of Foucault's words on the subject of the individual human being. He famously and contentiously proclaimed 'the end of man', arguing that the view of the human figure as the sovereign creator of meaning and experience is now 'in the process of disappearing' (1966, p. 420). Instead of crediting the person with the ability to stand as agent or cause of his or her life, an 'originator' of meaning, Foucault saw the individual as 'a variable and complex function of discourse' (1984, p. 118). As a function of discourse, which itself is inextricably tied up with social power dynamics, the individual is rendered 'the product of power' (1983, p. xiv); 'one of its prime effects' (1980c, p. 98). In other words, as human beings we are constituted by, and we are by-products of, the social power dynamics in which we live our lives.

Such understandings of the person are often celebrated by Foucauldian supporters as representing an advance over the naïve form of humanism that continues to shape so much of our thinking in the Western world (Falzon, 1998), according to which the individual is a sovereign, self-determining figure, who creates or authors himself or herself, as well as the world in which he or she lives. In a sense, Foucault reverses the image: the world creates the individual. As Paul Veyne notes, speaking of Foucault's vision:

> *What is made* [here, the individual as discursive subject]...is explained by what went into its *making* at each moment of history; we are wrong to imagine that the *making*, the practice, is explained on the basis of what is made.
>
> (Veyne, 1997, pp. 160–161)

By seeing the person as a product of the society and the time in which he or she lives, Foucault denies the individual the sovereign capacity to make the world in his or her own image, and according to his or her own desires. For supporters of Foucault, the significant advantage of this idea is that persons who are oppressed, marginalized, discriminated against, or even those who are dissatisfied with their lives, are no longer expected to simply pull themselves up by their bootstraps. Instead, Foucault usefully draws attention to the fact that it is power, social organization, and history – not the forces of personal choice, character, or willpower – that accounts for persons' locations in these disadvantaged positions. In this way he shows up the naïve individualism often associated with humanist discourse and its emphasis on living according to one's choices and free will.

But, in what Thiele (1990) has described as a 'remarkably uniform' debate, with two clear-cut and predictable positions being adopted (p. 907), other less sympathetic scholars took Foucault to task for precisely this stance. Yes, he highlights social power dynamics in a way that many humanist formulations obscure from view, but at what cost?

For many, he took too much away from the individual as such. Hall (2000) saw Foucault's reduction of the person to a discursive 'position' as a 'one-dimensional' vision (p. 23). And Jurgen Habermas – one of Foucault's most significant philosophical contemporaries, and in relation to whom Foucault has been described as a kind of 'wayward twin' (Conway, 1999, p. 76) – held that from Foucault's perspective, 'individuals can only be perceived as exemplars, as standardized products, of some discourse formation – as individual copies that are mechanically punched out' (1990, p. 293). Foucault's emphasis on power, for these readers, reduced the individual to whatever power and society told him or her to be. The individual, as such, seemed to be erased. Such critical readings of the Foucauldian human being, as a docile, manufactured puppet of power, are to be found in some measure in the works of numerous other scholars, such as Slavoj Žižek (2000), Nancy Fraser (1989), Charles Taylor (1986), and Edward Said (1986).

I list the names of these critics here for a rhetorical purpose: for some reason, many very clever people felt that Foucault did not make any theoretical room for a vision of the human being as an active, agentive figure who was capable of resisting power. Was he not killing off the individual as a social force in its own right? Indeed, Foucault's constitutionalist perspective of the person, which has been carried wholeheartedly into narrative practice (Freedman and Combs, 1996; White, 1993), is increasingly being seen as profoundly pessimistic (Heller, 1996), with critics bemoaning almost in single voice its apparent inability to allow for a cogent and coherent account of human agency and resistance.

It is worth noting that Foucault's sympathizers have responded to this agency critique, often arguing that there is more nuance in his work than such pessimistic readings suggest (e.g., Allen, 2000). Similarly, numerous defences refer to Foucault's emphasis on freedom, liberty, and resistance. From within the field of narrative therapy, Michael White expressed opposition to the view of Foucault as a 'philosopher of despair', and described, on the contrary, experiencing a 'special joy' when reading his work (2004, pp. 154–155). Clearly, White did not see the Foucauldian human being as a passive, docile figure. Others have argued that the pessimistic interpretations – even some of Foucault's own statements – are either misreadings or over-simplifications of his writing, particularly when looked at in the context of his overall body of works (e.g., Gutting, 1994; Heller, 1996; Veyne, 2010). What do his critics make of his call, in the years before his death, for us to 'create ourselves as a work of art' (Foucault, 1997c, p. 262)?

But let us, as narrative practitioners, hesitate before positioning ourselves in this debate (and we will explore aspects of the sympathetic interpretations in due course). In my opinion it would be a mistake to dismiss too quickly the thrust of the pessimistic readings; especially the concern that human agency and resistance are not clearly formulated in Foucault's works. There is *something* in this. And so I do not believe we should limit ourselves to thinking of Foucault's critics as either right or wrong. There is a third possibility, and it is this which stands as my point of departure: they point us towards a problem that is yet to be resolved.

We do not have to agree with Foucault's critics to note the importance of the challenge they lay down. And it is a challenge which is of profound relevance for the narrative practitioner. We have a question to answer: how are we to reconcile our Foucauldian constitutionalist perspective with our therapeutic vision of the person as imbued with personal agency, intentionality, and the capacity for resistance (e.g., White, 2007)? After all, characterizations of human beings as puppets, as 'mechanically punched out' effects of discourse, seem anathema to narrative therapy, replete as it is with optimistic accounts of the person. In our work, we orient to hearing stories of hope, of sparkling moments or unique outcomes, of preferred developments in people's lives, and of the personal agency linked to people's intentions, dreams, and values. Narrative therapy aims to assist in what White (2007) has referred to as the 'transporting' (p. 8) of persons towards hope, and aids in the generation of storied spaces – and, through these stories, personal and interpersonal spaces – through which life can be lived in preferred ways. As Freedman and Combs (1996) put it, we orient to 'the construction of an "agentive self" ' (p. 97). This is an optimistic, often solution-focused practice, following largely in the footsteps of that therapeutic optimist, Michael White.

So how do we reconcile the two stances we have given ourselves? How can the person exercise agency or resistance if he or she is a product of social discourses and power dynamics? And if not this, then who or what is the person?

Taking pessimism seriously

My goal here is not to try to guess what Foucault 'really meant'. For Gutting (1994), it would be naïve to expect some singular, unified answer in any case. Rather, our task is to use some of his ideas to help us understand and orient to the people who consult with us. And in this respect, the more pessimistic reading has something important to tell us.

Every therapist recognizes that there are times in persons' lives when a sense of agency, choice, freedom, and effective resistance seems absent, and when stuckness, paralysis, confusion, and powerlessness seem dominant. Almost every day we meet with people who experience aspects of their lives as hopelessly beyond their control. It is at these points that we might usefully think of the person as a product of social power dynamics; as a socially constituted subject. Such a formulation does not require a commitment to the view that this is all there is to the person. This, essentially, is the major criticism levelled at Foucault: his constituted subject is sometimes read as a total depiction of the person. It is clear that this was not Foucault's position, or perhaps following Gutting (1994) we should rather say that it was not his *only* position. Indeed, his close friend Paul Veyne (2010) says Foucault was horrified to hear that his work had been read in this way. I will not take up this debate at this point, except to say that the docile account is not one I will support here. Nonetheless, I suggest that in just some ways, in relation to certain issues, and with respect to certain problem-saturated experiences, the persons who consult with us may have been, or are being, socially shaped into forms that are powerfully capturing, unwanted, and which seem beyond their control.

And so while we might read Foucault's works in the joyful, optimistic ways that some of his apologists prefer – indeed, I will draw on certain interpretations of both Foucault and Nietzsche to try to justify a degree of optimism – I think it is significant that it is this same Foucault who can help us orient to and understand, not merely to overcome, the person's capture in power; his or her constraint in problem-saturated experience and identity. So I propose to begin our journey by taking seriously the pessimistic notion of the human being as a socially produced, constituted figure, even while accepting that there is more to the human being than this. I will put aside, but only temporarily, the question of human agency.

Having set this ground, I think we can say, without becoming members of the critical chorus, that in many of his works, Foucault (e.g., 1977) presented a rather bleak picture of the human being. But instead of rationalizing this away, we can see it as one of his most underappreciated (and inadvertent) contributions to our own therapeutic practices. He gave us a powerful series of demonstrations that personal freedoms and preferred developments can be very hard to come by. It would be too strong to say that narrative practitioners deny the difficulty people experience in trying to find some sense of personal agency. But the person's ineffectuality relative to the sometimes overwhelming nature of power, emphasized in Foucault's earlier works, seems to have been occluded in the narrative works inspired by him. We therapists might well acknowledge, name, and externalize experiences of powerlessness, fixedness, or stuckness (c.f., White, 2007), but we tend not to *examine* them, either theoretically or in the therapeutic relationship. The dominant narrative therapeutic practices – externalizing, re-membering, re-authoring, unique outcome development, witnessing – are geared far more towards the promotion of personal movement than towards understanding and exploring, for example, why movement and change can be hard to achieve, why people become stuck within problem-saturated stories, how people become attached to the labels imposed on them, why they stay with pain when it hurts them so much, or how they contribute to each other's and their own distress. These are not the aspects of human experience that we want to thicken, and so it is perhaps for this reason that there are no narrative therapeutic or conversational 'maps' of distress, emotional pain, or relationship breakdown.

So let us begin by looking at what the early Foucault showed us: the pessimism, despair, stuckness, paralysis, confinement, and control that people sometimes experience in their lives. And as we take seriously, and seek to better understand, the impact of the forces of social constitution on us and our identities, we will be better positioned to theorize and problematize – in a way that I believe is useful – the notion of personal agency, which has been so privileged in narrative practice. Our optimism is justified to the extent that we give it a cautious grounding: in power.

2
Power/Knowledge: The Social

In order to begin to conceptualize the human being, it is important to understand the dynamics of the social contexts in which people are constituted as subjects. As narrative therapists, who are in some measure constructionists, discourse analysts, and post-structural thinkers, we must begin our theoretical journey not with the individual, but with the social.

This might seem obvious, but we would do well to recall that, despite their theoretical convergences, Foucault and White oriented to different domains of human experience. Indeed, it is surprising in many respects that we would draw so heavily on Foucault, given that his work remains so easily transformable into one of the most devastating critiques of therapeutic practice we have available to us today. And so White (e.g., 2000, 2004), together with David Epston (e.g., White and Epston, 1990), performed an astonishing feat in making some version of Foucault's work *useful* for the therapeutic practitioner; and did so, moreover, without distorting or over-simplifying what Foucault found problematic about institutional practices such as psychotherapy. White and Epston found a way to work *with* Foucault, both to critique therapeutic practices, and to push these practices in directions that became increasingly sensitive to the issues of power and the related constitutive forces of sociality that so concerned Foucault. It might be useful to imagine White and Epston as explorers of the broad landscape painted by Foucault; as imaginers of how the individual might live, and be facilitated in living, in the social universe Foucault tried to describe.

Surely Foucault's biggest impact on narrative practice has occurred through his understanding of the social world in which the individual lives (Besley, 2002). This is a social world comprising rich, interconnected networks of power and knowledge. So strong is this interconnection that Foucault (1980a) referred to them in the form 'power/knowledge'. This conceptual amalgamation tells us that we cannot say what knowledge is without simultaneously working into our thinking some idea of the social conditions and power relations that are associated with this particular knowledge. Questions arise, such as: Who is entitled to perform this or that kind of knowing? Who is excluded from such knowledge practices? About whom does knowledge speak, and how are they constructed? What social hierarchies are supported by this or that knowledge? Who gains and who loses via this or that way of knowing? What other social 'work' is done with that knowledge? Knowledge, in other words, involves not just *knowing* but *doing*. Foucault put it this way: 'knowledge and power are integrated with each other... It is not possible', he maintained, 'for power to be exercised without knowledge, and it is impossible for knowledge not to engender power' (1980b, p. 52).

The power/knowledge nexus has been discussed at length in the narrative therapy literature (e.g., Besley, 2002; Madigan, 2011; White and Epston, 1990) and elsewhere (e.g., Rouse, 1994). I will not rehearse these discussions here, attempt to plot the development of Foucault's thought on this topic, or offer a step-by-step outline of each of his projects. Instead, my intention is to present aspects of the power/knowledge formulation that can help us orient to the person as a constituted subject, and which I have found useful in reflecting on my meetings with the people who consult with me. Once this context has been discussed, I turn in the following chapter to examine what it means to say that the individual is a constituted subject.

There are four aspects of power/knowledge that I wish to highlight: first, I will discuss how self-understanding is cultivated in a swarming array of knowledges; second, I consider how power operates through the forces of social alignment; third, I examine power's tendency to function as knowledge's invisible partner; and fourth, I touch on the view that discourses are intrinsically neither good nor bad. This is not intended as an exhaustive coverage of all that power/knowledge refers to, but it might nevertheless provide a useful platform for subsequent explorations of the person as a constituted subject, but also as one endowed with agentive potentials.

Cultivating self-understanding in a swarm of knowledge

In narrative practice people tell us stories about themselves and their worlds. The understandings conveyed by these stories are inevitably shaped by culturally available ways of knowing. For Foucault, our attachment to these specific knowledges reflects our inculcation into a broader 'will to knowledge' (1990a): a culturally and historically specific injunction that in order to live our lives properly, in socially synergistic ways, we should organize ourselves and our conduct around the truths or knowledges given to us, while simultaneously denying the social origins of those knowledges. That is, society demands that we account for ourselves in terms of the ways of knowing it provides, and act accordingly: as a man or a woman, black or white, child or adult, heterosexual or homosexual, normal or abnormal. But at the same time, we are given to understand that these are not socially constructed categories but 'natural' kinds of human being. In this section we will touch on the evolution of society's demand that we make ourselves known ('Who are you? What kind of person are you?') into its internalized form ('Who am I?') before focusing on how knowledge has become usable for the purpose of self-understanding, and how people's access to its multiplicity is constrained in the process.

Foucault's writings explored the ways in which, particularly from the nineteenth century onwards, knowledge became linked up with strategies of social control (e.g., 1979). Focusing initially on erudite, 'scientific discourse' centred on the subject of 'Man' (1980c, p. 84), he showed how disciplines like economics, criminology, psychiatry, and psychoanalysis set out not only to unveil the truths about the human being in general, but also to understand persons deemed troublesome: for example, criminals, the sick, the mad, wayward women and children, black persons, and homosexuals. It is as if society looked at such persons, and needed to know: 'Just who are you, and what can we do about you?' Such persons needed to be known so that they could be separated out, rendered predictable, and controlled (Mills, 2003). Far from being the neutral, objective practice it is popularly thought to be, knowledge became a tool with which to 'fix [these] useless or disturbed populations' and 'neutralize' the various 'dangers' they posed (Foucault, 1977, p. 210). Psychiatric and other knowledge forms articulated socially sanctioned truths about who such persons were, which in turn justified all manner of interventions, such as exclusion (e.g., the exclusion of black persons in apartheid South Africa; the incarceration of the mad), rehabilitation (e.g., the criminal), or cure (e.g., the naughty child, or the homosexual). Foucault's point is that knowledge came to function not as representation, but as intervention.

A good example of how this works is to be found in the historical relationship between psychoanalysis and human sexuality. For much of the twentieth century, many within this discipline promoted a stark division between heterosexuality and homosexuality. On the one hand, various theories were developed to 'explain' homosexuality as a deviant and psychopathological form of sexuality. Those identified as homosexuals became known (and in some circles continue to be known) in terms of all manner of fixations, projections, Oedipal conflicts, narcissistic identifications, and so on (e.g., Bergeret, 2002). In Foucauldian parlance, psychoanalysis helped entrench homosexuality not as a set of behaviours or preferences, but as a kind of identity. The homosexual was now a certain *type of person* – a type whose features could be identified by psychoanalysis – who had to be managed by being 'cured'. On the other hand, many psychoanalysts saw heterosexuality as indicative of a different type of person: a natural figure, whose 'normal' sexuality indicated successful parenting, and who represented the mature and healthy outcome of psychosexual development. These divisions, which reflected culturally and historically specific ways of understanding who the person was, and should be, were given shape, thickened with convincing scientific rationalities, and thereby produced as social realities, by such knowledge forms as psychoanalysis.

But the strategy of building objective knowledges about apparently disturbed or inconvenient populations, such as homosexuals, began to incorporate another strategy when these knowledges spread into the broader social domain: that of self-knowledge. Theoretically, this is a far more efficient strategy: instead of having the police, the courts, the experts, or the government control everybody from above, as it were, society could be better organized if people were recruited into, and thereby learned to see themselves and each other in terms of those knowledges: we should know and manage ourselves. 'A superb formula: power exercised continuously and for what turns out to be a minimal cost' (Foucault, 1980d, p. 155). For this localizing and internalizing move – from being known to knowing ourselves – to work, truthful discourses had to become more widely available and usable. Thus, the knowledges associated with disciplinary power – scientific wisdoms that aided in the management and control of certain populations – began to swarm. Foucault (1977) says they became 'de-institutionalized', emerging 'from the closed fortresses in which they once functioned ... to circulate in a "free" state' (p. 211). Knowledge could henceforth be used not merely by experts seeking to understand and manage 'useless or disturbed populations', but by everybody, to understand – and hence to manage – each other and themselves. Foucault (1977) put forward the Panopticon as a symbol of just such a shift. This architectural model exemplified the strategy of refining the management of persons: from surveillance by the authorities (e.g., prison guards, or for that matter, governments, parents, schoolteachers, doctors, therapists) to self-surveillance; a strategy that worked provided that people were inculcated into the proper norms and ways of knowing; provided they were properly constituted subjects.

It is no longer sufficient for governments, police, and so on, to govern us by fitting us into the right knowledge categories. Rather, the emphasis has shifted to self-governance. 'Who are you?' becomes 'Who am I?' Under the cultural and historical influence of the will to knowledge, we, the ordinary citizens, are aware that we cannot live properly if we do not know who we are; if we do not know, in unambiguous terms, our nationality, our race, our sexuality, our gender, our social class, our job profiles, our duties as parents, spouses, children, family therapists, and so on. There is often a price to pay for not knowing who one is (as a certain no-entry stamp on my passport attests). What is interesting, however, is that these categories of self-knowing are given to us, prescribed for us. This prescription allows for some semblance of mutual alignment in our self-knowing practices. The knowledge forms we share insure that we are all, in a sense, on the same page (as I shall discuss further below).

Thus, we have become 'subjects of knowledge' (Foucault, 1997c, p. 262); beings who must make sense of who we are in terms of the knowledge forms and categories available to us. These knowledges become so ingrained and taken-for-granted that we often use them to make conclusive judgements about ourselves and others. Take, for example, the wide circulation of psychoanalytic knowledges in certain societies. These knowledges continue to inform, sometimes as 'little moral narratives' (Parker, 2011, p. 6), common-sense thought and practice on such issues as childrearing, self-understanding, and sexuality. This widespread availability allows lay persons to engage in various kinds of self-observation, self-management, and moral judgement, in order to steer themselves in accordance with socially circulated, contextually adapted, psychoanalytic-like understandings. Lay and expert knowers alike can form psychoanalytically informed judgements of others: to label a neighbour as neurotic; a loved one as repressed; a homosexual as disturbed or perverted; to guess at who might or might not have had 'bad childhoods', etc. Disciplinary power – the informed, knowledge-based capacity, and perceived entitlement, to discipline ourselves and each other through acts of knowledge – has been 'disseminated throughout society' (Foucault, 1977, p. 212).

But we notice in our narrative practices that the self-understandings conveyed in our clients' stories are seldom so monolithic (e.g., in terms of a psychoanalytic view). The knowledges that Foucault tells us escaped from academia and other official sites, to circulate in 'a free state', do not spread as self-contained chunks of knowledge. Rather, the swarming of knowledge into the ordinary, non-expert social sphere is more often characterized by its adaptation, splitting, multiplication, and diversification. According to Foucault (1977), formal knowledges are 'broken down into flexible methods of control', and 'transferred and adapted' (p. 211) to suit various social circumstances. This malleability allowed such understandings to become linked up with a range of other knowledges – expert as well as religious, cultural, gendered, and other ways of knowing. So many knowledges have swarmed into our lives that a single human experience can easily be storied in multiple, often contradictory, ways. We witness this in the many and varied ways in which our clients understand themselves.

We are strongly attuned to the presence of multiple knowledges in narrative practice. But we should not then assume that persons are free to move around this multiplicity in coming to know themselves. There are at least two restraints to this freedom. First, social power relations open up some possibilities and close down others. How we know is always a hotly contested matter, which is always influenced by and further implicates relations of power. For example, in the case of homosexuality the stakes involved in answering the question can be very high. A person so labelled in the mid-twentieth century, for instance, would not be given much room to story his or her sexuality, nor even his or her identity, in personally preferred ways. This individual's attempts to portray himself or herself as 'normal' could result in various responses that powerfully undermine that intention. Official responses to such self-normalizations might have included disqualifying interpretations (e.g., 'you're in denial'), an intensified diagnosis (e.g., being seen as delusional), or the person might be incarcerated or even lobotomized. Multiple stories, and hence multiple ways of being a self, are always available in principle, but the consequences of inhabiting some of them can be serious indeed. Not all identities will do. And it is power, not truth, which determines which stories and identities will be accepted and seen as valid. So significant is this power that ways of knowing can determine who will lead and who will follow, who will find approval and who won't, who will be included and who excluded, and in some cases, who will live and who will die. In the case of homosexuality, then, social power dynamics would at certain historical points have pushed the person to answer the question – 'Who am I?' – in approved ways. For instance, the person might be encouraged to believe that he or she contained some 'natural' heterosexual core – the 'real me' – which, due to various traumas or other life events, were 'distorted' into homosexuality.

This brings us to the second impediment. The social requirement that we know ourselves means that we should pin ourselves to some specific self-understanding, and thereby self-limit our freedoms to move around this multiplicity. We should be disciplined in our self-understanding. The individual should 'be something': something recognizable, consistent, predictable even; something people can count on. For example, I might ask: Am I a good or a bad husband? A man or a woman? A soldier or a terrorist? A psychoanalyst or a narrative therapist? We are expected to have answers to such questions; fence-sitting is not highly valued. And so we see a narrowing down of the range of discourses that can be used for this purpose, while numerous other possibilities must be closed off. Of course, this identity-fixing can work to the person's advantage at times, to the extent that one finds oneself in a socially desirable position. But it can also be extremely limiting. We can become known, and know ourselves, in distressing ways, and also become trapped in identities that once served us well. At such times restricted access to other ways of being a person becomes especially problematic.

Let us take a therapeutic example to bring these issues closer to our specific concerns. Petra, a 26-year-old woman, came into therapy after her husband, Steve, left her for another woman just a month prior to our meeting, and one year into their marriage. She felt utterly lost and dejected, and could not find for herself a vision of a meaningful future. When I asked how this situation had arisen, she told me about her relationship with Steve, who she had always thought of as her 'Mr Right'. She told me about the first time they met some five years earlier, when they were both students at university. They were at a mutual friend's house when he approached her and they struck up a conversation. She immediately knew he was 'the one' for her, and felt that she had at last found her 'soul mate' after years marked by periods of loneliness alternating with disappointing and failed romances. She was reminded of something her father had once said to her: 'When you meet the right person, you just know.' It emerged as Petra and Steve got to know each other that they were born in the same town, that their families attended the same church, and that they went to the same nursery school, just one year apart. Several such coincidences added to Petra's sense of the inevitability of their coming together. This blissful story of the perfect couple continued on up to their wedding day, at which time she felt that

'God Himself' had blessed their 'union', and that the two of them 'had become one'. As she told this story to me, Petra explained how 'totally devastated' she was when she found out from a work colleague that her husband had been having an affair with one of her own friends. She reflected that she had gone from being 'a hopeless romantic' to feeling 'like my whole world was caving in, as if this is the end, there is no more'. She berated herself for 'being so stupid'.

The question here is: how should we understand Petra's situation with reference to the knowledge practices discussed above? As post-structural thinkers we reject the search for some internal, essential core (e.g., a psychological dynamic or process) that drives her behaviour from within. A psychiatrist had, some months earlier, diagnosed Petra with 'dependent personality disorder'. This label depicts an individual who depends on another for her well-being and self-definition, and who demonstrates extraordinary naiveté and gullibility (e.g., Millon, 1999). Despite the apparent fit of this description, there are several difficulties with it.

Because it builds from the inside out, such an account mislocates the social and cultural forces at play, and instead situates them within the person herself. It constructs Petra not as a person who in her lived experience answers the question of who she is in a particular set of ways – in ways which are shaped by the stories and discourses surrounding her; as a socially constructed figure – but simply as a person with a flawed kind of personality. As Foucault (1997d) might have put it, such a move confuses her cultural 'form' for an essential 'substance' (p. 290). In telling its own version of truth, this diagnostic discourse reinterprets those stories in which she is already constituted. Her stories of love, romance, and grief are thereby transformed into the personality characteristics of naiveté, gullibility, and a lack of independence. Instead of being seen as individual iterations of particular cultural ways of knowing and being, her stories simply signify a dependency at the core of her character. The diagnosis traps her in a tightly integrated, apparently truthful set of stories about her identity, such that the other multiple discourses that should, in principle, be available to her are effectively hidden or disqualified.

So instead of such an essentialist view of her 'personality' and its supposedly 'disordered' nature, let us think in terms of the infusion or swarming of knowledge into all corners of life. On that basis, we might better understand Petra's situation in terms of cultural knowledges that she has come to apply to herself in the form of a 'self-knowledge' as well as through the adoption of a kind of 'conscience' (in terms of how she feels she *should* live her life) (Foucault, 1982, p. 212). In this light we see her personal narratives not as reflections of internal disorder, but, in the

words of Michael White (2004), as 'carriers of culture'; each story serving as 'a vehicle for these (cultural) knowledges and practices' (p.
104), transporting them right into the intimate spaces of Petra's life.
We might notice, too, that Petra is held to these knowledges by both
forms of restraint discussed above. First, it seems Petra has become subject to widely circulated cultural and gendered knowledges which do not
simply offer but actively *prescribe*, and thereby limit, her ways of being:
that she should find herself, her happiness, and her very purpose in
life, in romance and marriage. Her compliance in this regard should not
come as a surprise, given that such knowledges are promoted in countless ways in the broader culture (e.g., in fairy tales, romance films and
novels, jewellery advertisements, etc.) (c.f., Burr, 1995). These knowledges link also with significant cultural institutions and practices, such
as religious ceremonies and ideals, which declare to the world that God
Himself has put these two persons together. In the context of this social
and cultural machinery, it might be difficult for Petra to meaningfully
situate herself in other stories of being.

And second, she self-limits her ways of knowing herself. Petra has
learned over time to hold herself to idyllic, romantic ways of thinking
about her life, and to discredit other ways of thinking and being which,
these romantic discourses tell her, are unromantic, unfulfilling, unfemi-
nine, or even masculine. This widely supported and decidedly gendered
romantic discourse seems to have powerfully influenced how she has
come to recognize who she is (or should be), and who she is not (or
should not be). The experiential thickness of these ways of knowing
makes it very difficult for Petra to access other narratives, despite their
presence in the broader culture. And so these romantic knowledges –
having swarmed across the social landscape; having divided up relational, social, and emotional tasks between men and women; having
been accelerated into different corners of people's hopes, fantasies,
and lives by various social, institutional, and media technologies and
practices; and having acquired a malleability enabling a diversity of
personalized applications – easily find a home in Petra's life.

Clearly, then, self-knowledge and social power dynamics are intimately related. But what precisely do we mean by power?

Power as productive social alignment

The spread of any particular knowledge form (such as that of romance)
throughout society is not sufficient to give it such power in a person's
life. The widely circulated existence of a way of knowing does not in

itself guarantee that it will become influential in shaping our sense of self. Knowledge must be grafted onto power relations to have such an effect.

Let us quickly clarify what power is not. Power does not, in Foucault's work, point to the individual, and his or her capacities. It is not 'a certain strength we are endowed with' (Foucault, 1990a, p. 94); it is not something a person possesses or does not possess. We cannot say, for instance, that Petra has been robbed of power, as if it were something she once possessed but which was seized by her husband. Rather, power is always a social, relational phenomenon. 'The term "power" ', says Foucault, 'designates relationships between partners' (1982, p. 217), and does not exist except as power *relations*.

We can think of power in terms of the alignment of social practice with the structures and dictates of particular discourses (Rouse, 1994; Wartenburg, 1990). In other words, power refers to the social and institutional *coordination* required to produce and introduce elements of knowledge into social reality; a set of diverse communal forces which come together to enforce the actualization, the coming true, of knowledge. For example, Petra's position as a disappointed romantic is part of a more or less socially coordinated network of behaviours, attitudes, beliefs, and socially circulated stories and practices about romance, in which she participates. We might wonder if she has been recruited into this discourse as a romantic subject. And to the extent that she has, she thereby becomes part of, and a player in, the socially and culturally coordinated performance of romance.

How was Petra recruited into this place? We cannot answer such a question in anything like a comprehensive way, but Petra told me of some events and memories that might have contributed to her sense that this was the right way to be. She recalled, for instance, as a young girl pretending to dress up as a bride. Also, after certain romantic disappointments during her adolescence, her parents would often tell her that she just hadn't found 'Mr Right' yet. She also told me about certain films and novels that depicted a range of romantic relationships, all of which contributed to a sense that her desire to find this elusive man was perfectly natural. These events involve a complex web of relationships (e.g., with her parents and peers), cultural practices (e.g., films, novels) and institutions (e.g., the wedding, marriage), which more or less aligned to lure her from an early age towards the promises of romance. We can think of these relationships, practices, and institutions as loosely coordinated social elements which functioned – via their alignment – to bring romance to life, to make it real, and to make it a place of potential belonging and self-recognition for Petra.

This coordination of social activities shows also, as Foucault (e.g., 1980a) argued, that power tends to be productive rather than repressive in its tactics. Power positively transforms us into, shapes or constitutes us as, 'appropriate' social actors. For instance, the power of romantic discourse lies not only in its repression or downgrading of certain alternative positions, roles, or duties. Certainly, negative depictions of lonely, childless spinsters might be useful in supporting the cultural idealization of romantic discourse. But if this was all that power did (and again I am thinking of power as institutionally and socially coordinated action) – work negatively, saying no to, and steering us away from what it deemed undesirable – it could not, except perhaps through chance, produce the sort of world its discourses describe. Rather, power works by constructing and nudging us towards its ideals; by making certain positions attractive. Its effectiveness rests on its capacity to actively recruit people into becoming subjects who willingly and appropriately play this particular social game, and make sense of themselves, their thoughts, actions, and feelings accordingly. Power strives to provoke conduct that is appropriate to the discourses it operates through.

Thus, societal coordinations around romantic discourse do not explicitly aim to *remove* Petra's sense of independence or competence (i.e., which might be consistent with a view of power as negative or repressive), but instead move to *make her* romantic, trusting, loving, and so on (i.e., power as positive). Petra is produced, not repressed, into a romantic subject.

Repression is not an efficient strategy because, first, it does not necessarily lead to the positive human forms that power requires. For instance, any overt crushing or repression of Petra's sense of personal agency and autonomy would not automatically turn her, specifically, into a romantic subject. A range of responses are available to the crushed person: depression, withdrawal, suicide, fighting back, and, perhaps, clinging to another in romance. A repressive strategy could hardly be counted on to lead specifically to the last of these outcomes.

Second, as Foucault (1980d) noted, nakedly repressive tactics tend to provoke resistance: 'If power were never anything but repressive, if it never did anything but to say no, do you really think one would be brought to obey it?' (p. 119) Refusal is often an inconvenience from the perspective of power (although we shall see later that it can also be a useful stimulus for power's evolution). Indeed, Petra would be far more likely to resist power if she was explicitly required to be docile – if she was told in so many words that her life was to be one of service to a man, that she should sacrifice her own needs and desires, and define herself only in terms of that relationship – than if her docility was constructed in terms of a valuable place within, and through the magical promises of, love and romance. Power relies on a picture being painted by the knowledge forms with which it is associated. Docility can then be constructed in more appealing feminine terms: it is not that Petra is oppressed or silenced, but that she is gentle, kind, unassuming. Romantic discourse works most effectively not if Petra feels squashed, but if she is positively sold on romance; if she is persuaded through life experience that it is good, rewarding, pleasant, and meaningful to participate in those kinds of relational games; if she perceives what Althusser (1971/2008) termed an 'obviousness' about such a way of being in the world.

To take another example: Petra's tendency to defer to the apparent wisdom of her husband is not simply a matter of the erosion of her self-confidence, or of her dependency (in her psychiatrist's view), but the positive form made available to her by a particular social power game of romance. Her deference, that is, far from representing the suppression of self-expression and meaning, comes to contain its own rich meanings, promises, and values, supported by a wealth of historical experience. It becomes, in a sense, part of her way of being in the world. Deference might contribute to a certain style of appealing femininity, in the context of heterosexual romantic relationships. Her deference allows her to find a positive position for herself within complex socially coordinated activities around romance and related stories and practices, which in turn make her recognizable to herself and to others in a particular way. Of course, given the multiplicity of human experience, we are likely to notice that sometimes Petra slips away from, or even protests against, such ways of being, despite the appealing constructions associated with them. But we will come to such matters later on.

For now, we note that power 'incites, it induces, it seduces' (Foucault, 1982, p. 220). It makes some things easier (e.g., for Petra to be demure, deferring, gullible, naïve, and supportive of the needs of the other), and other things more difficult (e.g., for her to be assertive and expressive of her own needs). In such ways, power is able to generate the characters and other elements needed for romance stories to come to life; to become socially real. And it achieves this through complex webs of socially coordinated human activity.

The idea that power tends to be subtly productive rather than nakedly repressive suggests that there is something underhanded about it. Indeed, power is frequently invisible.

Power is knowledge's invisible partner

Before commenting on power's relative invisibility in the power/ knowledge relationship, I want to say something about the mutual productivity that pertains between these two aspects of discourse: knowledge and power work together to produce and reproduce each other.

On the one hand, knowledge produces power relations, in the sense that it defines activities, social roles, and personal positions for designated persons (e.g., psychiatric patient, psychiatrist, nurse, in the context of psychiatric knowledges; or the various gendered positions around discourses of romance), and thereby constructs coordinated systems of power relations. Knowledge explicitly or implicitly tells social participants what to expect, how to behave, what their entitlements are, whose opinions should hold sway under which circumstances, and so on. Power emerges within socially coordinated activities, as social actors hold each other to knowledge-prescribed positions and behaviours, and press for mutual compliance.

But, on the other hand, knowledge can also be built on a platform provided by already existing power relations. For example, when therapist and client meet there is a pre-structured power relation already in place, produced by (among other things) over a century of professional and cultural discourse about therapeutic practice. This structures a particular form of social coordination in terms of which therapist and client orient to each other. One result of this is that a particular power arrangement is set up in the room before therapist and client even meet. Among other things, this lends a sort of gravity to the therapist's beliefs and judgements that the client cannot easily match. As family therapist Carl Whitaker said, 'We put people in hospital because they have delusions. If I have a delusion they call it a theory' (1982, p. 368). The therapist's and client's knowledges have different statuses because they operate on the basis of an already existing power relationship, which is accepted in and supported by the broader culture. In other words, a fixed power dynamic can pre-date certain specific social interactions, thereby predetermining who can produce knowledge, and of what kind.

So power and knowledge are intimately linked, but they differ in terms of their empirical accessibility. Knowledge tends to be accessible and explicit, while the workings of power are often more difficult to pinpoint. According to Foucault (1988b), 'relations of power are perhaps among the best hidden things in the social body' (p. 118). Power is the silent one, the hidden one, in this partnership.

What does this mean? I want to address four broad interrelated aspects of power's concealment, so that we might better appreciate the unseen ways in which power shapes the ways in which we know ourselves: first, discourse produces stories and practices that obscure from view the orchestration of social activities required for its maintenance and effects; second, a successful discourse conceals alternative ways of knowing and doing; third, much discourse turns our attention away from power in order to illuminate the person instead; and fourth, discourse is sometimes naturalized, coming to seem self-evidently true.

Discourse is underpinned by an invisible ensemble of social practices

If power refers to the social coordination of activities that maintain a particular discourse, then it will work best, and prevent meaningful resistance, when key aspects of this social orchestration are hidden from view.

To illustrate the depth of this invisibility, and the contribution it can make to the maintenance of a particular identity, let us think through Whitaker's distinction between the theory-producing therapist and the delusion-generating client. Whitaker's tongue-in-cheek remark speaks to the cultural and historical privileging of the 'psy complex' in making sense of personal phenomena, especially in the Western world (Ingleby, 1985; Rose, 1985). This complex refers to a range of interrelated practices, led by culturally designated professionals, such as the psychologist, psychiatrist, psychoanalyst, and psychotherapist: the psy practitioners. These professionals are positioned as expert knowers in a way that their clients and the rest of the population cannot hope to match. The distinction between the knowing therapist and the not-knowing client is often given a sound rationale, which 'everybody' knows and which seems hardly worth mentioning. Many enculturated persons, for instance, are equipped to reasonably argue that the therapist is trained in neutral, truth-generating scientific methods, while the client's judgement is not only inferior because it is informed by lay and common-sense knowledges, but is also likely clouded by his or her mental health difficulties. This very ordinary, seemingly self-evident rationale for privileging the therapist's words and actions underpins several therapeutic practices which rely on this systematic therapist-client differentiation. Consider the therapist's declaration of a diagnosis, the deployment of transference interpretations in psychoanalysis, and the identification of negative automatic thoughts and core beliefs in cognitive behavioural therapy: all of these practices rely on the therapist being credited with special powers of knowledge, discernment, and judge-ment. Narrative practitioners are not immune from the effects of such ways of thinking, insofar as we are subsumed in a wider network of meanings and subject to common sense discourse about therapy and therapists. Thus, regardless of our collaborative intentions, some clients easily position us as expert knowers, and might well resist our efforts to decentre our own position (c.f., Young, Saunders, Prentice et al., 1997).

So, cultural stories are available to explain and justify the therapist's status as expert knower. But much is concealed by those discourses. Specifically, it can be hard to see the considerable and wide-ranging social activity that sustains this way of understanding the therapist's position relative to his or her client. Whitaker's therapeutic knowledge could not work in the way that it does were it not for the coming together of innumerable social and historical factors that press for his delusion to be called a theory, and for the client's theory to be called a delusion. Whitaker recognizes that he does not achieve therapeutic cleverness by himself. He has considerable, but invisible, assistance.

For one thing, he already tells us that others interpret his crazy, delu-sional words as organized, clever, 'theory'. But there are many additional factors, some rather distal, that support him in this regard. His affili-ation to a professional therapeutic association gives him professional and legal status, lends his words a certain gravitas, and allows him to put certificates on his office walls. His explicit and implicit links with psychiatrists, doctors, psychologists, lawyers, and insurance companies serve to authorize his pronouncements. Indeed, these persons and insti-tutions stand as a veritable army, waiting to act should he deem it necessary. The 'Carl Whitaker' reputation, circulated among family ther-apy circles in particular, no doubt assists in the meaning and weighting people find in and attribute to his words. We like to have therapeu-tic heroes, and so Whitaker's reputation allows him to be turned from human being into something more: a symbol, an embodiment of thera-peutic wisdom. He has become one of our gurus. And so we incorporate some element of panache into our stories of his practices: his play with a handkerchief in a session is not 'unconventional', as it might be seen were he a novice or unknown therapist, but 'genius'. Even people who don't know him are nudged to invest his words with wisdom. The por-trayal of other therapists, psychiatrists, and psychologists in movies, books, talk shows, and newspaper and magazine reports, lead to some-thing like his form of talk and style of interaction circulating through society, so that when he meets his clients they have learned how to orient to him in an 'appropriate' way. They all know, in some measure, to treat, to *interpret*, his delusions as clever theories.

But our construction of Whitaker as a therapeutic hero has support from sources that might make us more uncomfortable. Kendall and Wickham (1999) note that powerful discourses are very often built on 'disreputable origins and unpalatable functions', rather than on neutral academic or scientific discoveries (p. 34). One of the things that no doubt assists Whitaker's reputation – and that of all of us in the therapeutic professions – is the disqualification of common-sense wisdoms and other local knowledges (c.f., Foucault, 1980c). Kitzinger and Perkins (1993) argue, from a feminist perspective, that this has led to the undermining of trust within local communities, increasingly prompting people to turn away from the experienced, wise advisers they might once have consulted within their own communities, and instead to seek out the designated psychological truth tellers, such as psychologists and psychotherapists. Worryingly, it seems that such deferral to the experts is on the increase. Psychiatric diagnostic systems, such as the 5th edition of the *Diagnostic and Statistical Manual of Mental Disorders*, are increasingly being constructed in such a way that more and more people qualify for diagnoses (Frances, 2010). This carries the implication that more and more people will be beyond the reach of common-sense knowers and helpers. The counsel of wise family members, friends, and traditional healers loses value. In a sense, Whitaker's success (and our own) builds on such systematic, though largely invisible, disqualifications of a host of non-professional voices.

I use this example to demonstrate that the concealment of the emergent coordination of a very wide range of social activities allows a discourse to succeed, to become powerful and influential, as if on its own merits. In our case, we note that such invisibilization helps sustain therapeutic discourse itself, and allows its practitioners' voices to be valorized. Power is invisible insofar as the coordination of these wide-ranging sociocultural activities is seen not as the strategic achievement of a particular set of discourses, or as the product of complex struggles between extant ways of knowing and doing, but as the neutral, impartial, taken-for-granted, 'natural' hustle and bustle of social activity. It seems self-evident that our expertise is intrinsically superior, and that community members once considered wise have at last been exposed for their lack of expert, scientific knowledge; it is just 'the way things are'. The result is that Whitaker is often seen as a genius, while the vast network of supporting cast, props, and activities, including the silencing and demotion of figures once credited with significant therapeutic-like wisdom, goes unnoticed.

I want to mention that, of course, the individual can develop considerable skills through his or her embodiment in, and practice of discourse. And, as we shall see, I do not suggest that the individual is no more than the positions to which he or she is assigned by discourse. Carl Whitaker was indeed a very clever therapist! But his brief statement concerning the cultural valorization of his delusions seems to point to his awareness that he was powerfully assisted by an entire ensemble of virtually invisible social partners.

Any identity ascription – genius, loser, schizophrenic – rests on some such degree of invisibilization.

The concealment of alternative discourses

I alluded above to the idea that power often works via the disqualification or downgrading of other ways of knowing and doing. This includes, but is not limited to, local, folk, common-sense, and other forgotten knowledges, which somehow do not meet the threshold of cleverness required for them to be valued in particular socio-cultural locales. But there are also other erudite, well-articulated, sometimes even 'scientifically' supported knowledges, which can be dismissed or downplayed. The social alignment of activities which serve a particular discourse can function to make even well-thought out and academically developed ways of knowing, such as feminist knowledges (as we shall see below), seem inferior, naïve, unworkable, distasteful, or they might even conceal them altogether.

Let us return to Petra's situation of being positioned in a discourse of romance. There has been much theoretical and empirical attention to the stories and practices of romance. Some of this work has the potential to bring to light some of the otherwise hidden power tactics associated with romance. For example, in her discussions on social constructionism, Vivienne Burr (1995) argued that discourses of romantic love 'mask inequitable social arrangements', such as the expectation that women provide a range of 'services free of charge', including taking care of meals, children, upkeep of the home, and so on (pp. 72–73). According to Burr, this discourse constructs marriage in a way that obscures both men's and women's visions of such social conditions. The idea here is that common Western notions of romantic love often cloud our view of the disadvantaged position women can find themselves in in heterosexual partnerships, while simultaneously making these relationships seem desirable; indeed, the very route to self-fulfilment. Some have argued that such idealizing discourses encourage women to construct their whole identities around their relationship with a particular man, in a way that is not required of their male partners (Naffine, 1994).

But before wholeheartedly accepting these persuasive remarks, I think we should question Burr's use of the term 'mask' as a way of characterizing the relationship between romance and gender inequality. As post-structural thinkers, we need to be cautious about assuming that there is some objective reality out there (e.g., unequal gender power relations), on the one hand, and discourses which represent this reality either accurately (e.g., Burr's theory) or inaccurately (e.g., Petra's romance stories), on the other. As Dreyfus and Rabinow (1982) maintain: 'The world is not a play which simply masks a truer reality that exists behind the scenes' (p. 109).

I do not assume this is where Burr is coming from, but it is interesting to note that the classical Marxist reading of power, aspects of which continue to shape the way we think about that issue (Heller, 1996), particularly in the Western world, promotes precisely this kind of distinction. Burr's idea that romance 'masks' the real social conditions of gender inequality reminds me of such a perspective. I do not pretend to offer a comprehensive account of the Marxist position here, but a brief discussion might help clarify what it is that power conceals or 'masks' from us (e.g., in the case of romance), and to distinguish a classical Marxist account from a Foucauldian understanding.

On the classical Marxist account, power operates via ideologically orchestrated 'false consciousness' (Engels, 1893) – a term which, it seems, was not used by Marx himself (Eagleton, 1991) – in the service of capital, and its small number of beneficiaries. To begin with, power draws us into a palatable, if not sometimes beautifully painted picture. The contents of this picture might concern any number of cultural institutions and ideals. For example, we might see religion as the route to our salvation; we might approve of a therapeutic approach because it is collaborative; and we might buy into the wonderful promises of romance. But for many in the classical Marxist tradition, these stories serve ideological purposes: our belief in them has us unwittingly serving the interests of a select and powerful few. This is why it is termed false consciousness: we are not aware of, or we misrecognize, the true nature of our beliefs and actions. 'In ideology', says Engels, 'men and their circumstances appear up-side down as in a camera obscura' (Marx and Engels, 1974, p. 47). On this account, we have been seduced into serving power, while our ideologically shaped beliefs blind us to the more exploitative truth: that religion is the 'opiate of the masses' and impedes political rebellion; that the notion of collaborative therapy usefully masks therapeutic manipulations and serves the entire psy complex and its professional class; and that illusions of romance conceal gender inequality and thereby protect the male class from criticism and keep them in a privileged position.

We should note at this point that Marxist and post-Marxist theory is a complex field, in which thought has developed beyond the simplistic view of false consciousness and ideology described above (e.g., Eagleton, 1991). Nevertheless, these kinds of ideas continue to shape common-sense and much other thinking on power. So my aim here is to highlight these issues in general terms in order to lend clarity to my understandings of discourse and power.

It is interesting, then, to note that the notion of ideology continues to be used in much of the theorizing around narrative practice, for instance as a way of understanding the link between 'social ideas and politics, power, and practices' (Madigan, 2011, p. 58). But there are reasons to be cautious. From a Foucauldian perspective, it is misleading to think of the masking tactics of discourse (e.g., of gender inequalities) in terms of the classical Marxist version of ideology. First, the twin notions of ideology and false consciousness rest on a discursively untenable 'truth/falsity' distinction (Purvis and Hunt, 1993, p. 479); a distinction which issues from a representational rather than constructive or productive view of discourse. And second, these notions assume the existence of some master class of persons (capitalists, psychologists, men), who somehow stand above subjectification, author the subservience of others, and reap the rewards of their exploitation. Rather, Foucault (1980d) tells us, power is more like 'a machine in which everyone is caught, those who exercise power just as much as those over whom it is exercised' (p. 156). Taking these two points then, Petra's belief in romance should not be seen in terms of her positioning in a false story which hides or masks the truth (a kind of false consciousness), and neither her husband nor men in general should be treated as the strategic Machiavellian beneficiaries.

Of course, Burr is right that there is some concealment of power relations at play here. What is hidden, though, is not some objectively true state of affairs, as if there were some true discourse we could use to unveil reality itself. Rather, it becomes harder to see other culturally available ways of thinking about, organizing, and performing gender or other kinds of relationships. Discourses can only obscure other discourses; not objective truth. Among these other ways of thinking about and performing gender are the discourses of inequality to which Burr refers, and a host of other ways of thinking about gender relations. These concealed or marginalized discourses are useful, not because they are more true or inherently 'better' than that of romance (and we should be careful not to essentialize gender as somehow more real than other discourses and discursive effects), but because they help to disrupt the hegemonic effects of a prevailing state of affairs: in this instance, romantic discourse. Among the multiple effects of romance discourse may be its tendency to produce women who provide home services 'free of charge', as Burr puts it (1995, p. 73), and women whose identities depend on their male partners (Naffine, 1994). But these too are stories, and we do not undermine the importance of challenging masculine hegemony if we insist on that. We should note that Petra, and many others, might reasonably give a different account of this discourse's effects, including feelings of security and belonging, and its promotion of an ethic of care for the other. So when we say that a discourse (e.g., romance) has real effects in the social world we must remember that these effects cannot be neutrally or objectively observed and described. They too are subject to the requirements of discourse; they must be storied in order to have any meaning for us, and if they are to call us to action when it seems options for living are being closed down.

So, with respect to Burr's and others' discourses about romance masking inequality, the question here shifts from, 'How is this unequal reality concealed?' to 'How are these resistance-provoking *discourses and possibilities for action* concealed, minimized, or disqualified?' A small shift, perhaps, but an important one nonetheless. It helps us to avoid reifying one version of reality and affirming that story's values and associated practices. It prevents us from assuming an entitlement to impose our own understandings of reality on the persons with whom we work.

Cultural discourses – widely circulated truths, taken up in socially aligned ways – prompt us to story things in some ways rather than others (e.g., in terms of romance), and to overlook or downplay some of the effects of that discourse. I suggest that Petra's life narratives are such that the discourses of gender equality and associated practices, such as those suggested by Burr, are not well articulated and storied, and hence seem unworkable. There might seem to be few points in her life onto which they can become 'hooked', and take on significance. They do not feel grounded in her life. And in contrast to the thickened network of social practices and cultural stories that align to support romance, the social, institutional, and narrative supports for ideas concerning gender equality/inequality are not so strong in Petra's life history. All of this points to a kind of concealment of the discourses of gender equality. However, this does not necessarily amount to their total invisibility.

Petra is not blind to these alternatives, but she seems to have access to only a thin, somehow unrelatable and unworkable, description of these narratives and practices. She demonstrated her awareness of some of these ideas when she answered some of my questions (about why it might have been easier for her husband than for her to move on) by saying, quite unapologetically: 'But I'm not a feminist!' I think she cannot feel herself a feminist because these more questioning and resisting knowledges, which cast a critical eye on gender dynamics, seem to lack substance in her experience as a romantically constituted subject. What is concealed is the thickness, the habitability, of other ways of knowing.

Individualization: Discourse illuminates the person, not power

The tactics of individualization and internalization make it difficult for persons to recognize the extent of the social practices on which the constituting discourse relies. According to Foucault, modern power functions to make the person visible in order to conceal itself: 'In discipline it is the subjects who have to be seen', not power (1977, p. 187).

In order to achieve this, modern discourse often promotes a view of the person's experience as 'caused' by internal, individual factors. This is no doubt supported by the idealization of self-contained individualism in the Western world (Sampson, 1993). Among other things, the cultural story of this individual is of one who is self-determining and takes personal responsibility for his or her actions and circumstances. It is easy to see how such a valorization of individualism leads to the idea that we should, in order to appear competent or adult, locate the cause of our actions within ourselves. Likewise, personal deficiencies or weakness should also be attributed to internal process, while the social factors involved in such characterizations are overlooked.

Over the last century in particular, the psy discourses entrenched this internalizing tendency, pushing people to understand their lives in terms of individual behaviours, attitudes, beliefs, and choices; in terms of their psychological make-up. Cushman (1995) suggests that this tendency gathered further momentum after World War II, in the form of a 'preoccupation with "the self", its natural qualities, its growth, its "potential", abstracted out of and removed from the sociopolitical' (p. 240). Individualism, he adds, was 'elevated to an unquestioned social value' (p. 240). This proved to be an enabling environment for the humanistic movement in psychology – or rather, Cushman suggests, a 'decidedly apolitical' version of humanism (p. 242) – which incorporated, among other things, an emphasis on 'such distinctively human qualities as choice, valuation, and self-realization', and 'an interest in the development of the potential human inherent in every person' (pp. 240–241).

From the perspective of narrative practice, this energized spread of humanism at that time is of some interest. The humanistic tradition stands as the exemplar of the kind of decontextualized thought and practice that narrative therapists contest. Above all others, it is *the* discourse that explicitly shines its light on the person rather than power. In the process it constructs what is – from our perspective – a naïve view of human agency, associated with such notions as free will, choice, personal growth, and the release of the individual's inner 'potential'. These are the very concepts that we problematize, as they seem to overlook the constitutive forces associated with power/knowledge, and thereby render invisible the operations of power that shape the person's identity and ways of being. Little wonder then that humanism is the form of thought with which, against which, Foucault struggled for much of his working life (Falzon, 1998).

The idealization of self-contained individualism; the emergence of the psy complex and its army of practitioners; the fine-tuned discourses of humanism and its spread into multiple areas of our lives: such developments facilitated a focus on the individual as the sole cause of his or her life experience. David Epston (1993) referred to those discourses that promote this inward focus as 'internalizing discourses' (p. 161). These discourses easily cast a shadow over social, economic, or cultural factors. And the invocation of such factors as ways of accounting for persons' failures to measure up to the standards of success prescribed for them can be branded as excuses. One's life potential, the internalizing discourse declares, is in one's own hands. Economic conditions and prejudicial practices are thereby downgraded as explanatory factors, and may even come to seem irrelevant to the life circumstances in which a person finds himself or herself.

I find it useful to think of individualization and internalization in terms of the swarming of discourse into the intimate areas of our lives. The achievement of the internalizing discourses that Epston refers to is not merely that we shape our identities out of the cultural stories and ideals, values, and norms that surround us, but that we simultaneously deny their socio-cultural origins. Individualization requires that we should not see the power relations implicated in the forging of the stories and values that seem to become our own. And we should not see the downgrading of other knowledges, or the processes by which certain persons' voices are disqualified or diminished.

Sampson (1993) suggests that such invisibility attends every characterization of oneself, whether in preferred terms or not. In his articulations of self-contained individualism, he highlights that the maintenance of a particular and culturally preferred identity (e.g., as 'calm and rational'; as 'organized') rests on the – at least implicit – construction of others in devalued ways (e.g., as 'emotional'; as 'disorganized or crazy'). Likewise, negative identity conclusions (e.g., 'I am a loser') rest on the at least implicit recognition of others with more positively valued identities (e.g., 'winners'). For Sampson (1993), the person installed in the negatively valued position is a 'serviceable other', or a 'hidden dialogic partner' (p. 19), without whom the instalment of others in more desirable, successful, or valued positions would not be possible. One cannot say what one is without at least implicitly constructing the other in some kind of contrasting position, which lends meaning to the former. Narrative analyst Michael Bamberg (e.g., 2004) has also usefully noted the reverse: one cannot say what *another* person is without at least implicitly constructing *oneself* in some way.

Sampson tells us that these kinds of interactional processes help maintain particular identities, even as they are themselves concealed by individualizing discourses. We must remember that, from a Foucauldian perspective, such relational ascriptions are only possible because of the widespread availability and privileging of certain cultural knowledges, in terms of which (for example) rationality is deemed better than emotionality; in terms of which competition is valued, meaning in turn that winning is better than losing. Under the influence of individualism, particularly in the West (Geertz, 1979; Sampson, 1993), such cultural knowledges and value systems are internalized. Individualization not only conceals our relationality, as Gergen (1999) notes, but obscures also the cultural forms and value systems that define the terms – the contents – for the structuring of those relationships.

It is one thing to note that internalizing discourses are underpinned by unseen social forces. But, perhaps by now for obvious reasons, the person hardly experiences his or her sense of self as socially produced. The individualizing trend of much modern discourse is so effective that we often experience internalized cultural knowledges as personally meaningful, even as of our own making. They feel intimately part of who we are; as if they have welled up from deep within us, so powerful is their stamp on our personal meaning-making. Lock and his colleagues (2005) suggest that one of the functions of narrative therapy is to make visible these invisible social forces. But this can be a very difficult therapeutic task. Sometimes, in my experience, persons feel that talk about the socio-cultural stories and practices that recruited them misses the mark: 'No, it's not out there, it's in here!' This is testament to the power of individualization.

A 23-year-old university student, Tholani, seeking help for his 'anxiety' and 'constant worrying', told me about the time, at 13 years of age, when he overheard his mother, a psychiatric nurse, telling a neighbour: 'Tholani is a worrier.' He told me: 'That really stuck in my brain, and I still remember it so clearly.' We should note, however, that Tholani's father had been an anti-Apartheid activist in the late 1980s in South Africa, in the final years of that political system. Under the State of Emergency that was in place at the time, police could arrest activists quite freely, and many were beaten and sometimes even killed. This was the dangerous world in which Tholani and his family lived. His mother made the comment about Tholani being a 'worrier' around this time; at a time in which his father was at significant risk. For me, as a narrative practitioner, it seemed obvious that in terms of Tholani's experience of himself as a worrier, there were ample recruitment events present in his life, from his mother's declaration of his anxious psychological traits, through to the vulnerable position he and his family, and especially his father, were in with regard to the police and the Apartheid system. Indeed, as a young teenager Tholani spent many sleepless nights worrying about his father's safety. It seemed to me there was an entire social universe calling Tholani into worry.

But what struck me was how he saw all of these events as merely triggers for his pre-existing inclination to worry. So deep, so thick, was this sense of himself, that it was as if his mother had simply recognized a 'fact' about his psychological nature. His mother, in her recirculation of discursively available wisdoms (something we all do), had assigned him a culturally suitable category of personhood, and, apparently, Tholani found himself well represented in this story. Understandably, he interpreted surrounding events as some of the multiple sites in which his a priori tendency to anxiety was exposed; and his mother's account not as a convenient, ready-to-hand, and decontextualized narrative – one of many possible culturally available understandings – but as her recognition of his true self. 'She knew me so well. I've always been a worrier', he said. This sense of himself did not feel in any way imposed on him, or authored for him by some wider set of discourses and practices. Any hint of this kind of talk on my part seemed to bring about disengagement. In these moments, it must have seemed to him that I did not understand that worrying was simply 'core' to his personhood.

Petra, after losing her husband to another woman, also internalized the experience, speaking of herself as 'stupid' for having put herself in this position of vulnerability in the context of her romantic relationship in the first place. But in terms of the perspective articulated here, we know that this vulnerability is sponsored by cultural discourses that Petra had no hand in constructing, but which had recruited her into their practices. Such internalizing descriptions as 'stupid' and 'dependent personality disorder' have us looking for understanding in all the wrong places. We hear Petra critiquing herself as stupid, but as narrative practitioners we would instead like to pose questions about the multiple ways in which she – and millions of others – have been successfully pulled into the performance of such cultural narratives. In other words, we externalize rather than internalize the issue in our thinking, and thereby highlight rather than conceal the impact of social power dynamics.

Both Tholani and Petra construct their experience such that the light of discourse, to paraphrase Foucault, does not shine on the multiple ways in which their situations have been constructed and reproduced, but on their 'selves'; on Tholani's worrying nature, and Petra's stupidity and dependency. The person is visible, not power.

Naturalization: 'It's just the way it is'

The final point I wish to make about power serving as knowledge's invisible partner is this: the construction of particular human experiences as 'natural' can make the interpersonal dynamics of a situation seem like expressions of 'the way things are'. These are the taken-for-granted assumptions that Foucault suggests become so embedded in our thinking that we cannot see any way around them (Veyne, 2010).

Thinking once more of Petra's situation, it is evident that in much of the Western world, romantic love is considered 'a "natural" feature of human nature' (Burr, 1995, p. 72). For Petra, in fact, her experience was even more than this; it was a process blessed by God. Such a belief in a divine structuring of one's life makes it extremely difficult to appreciate the possibility of alternative understandings. Indeed, this naturalized, even God-given, status of romance discourse might promote even further self-criticism in a situation such as Petra's. For instance, it might push her to question herself: Did she listen to God in the right way? Did she perhaps do something to deserve the loss of her man? Did God send her warnings about Steve that she did not listen to? What if Steve really is her soul mate after all, and this is a test of their love? Self-questioning makes sense in this context because, after all, error cannot lie in a divine, natural, and self-evident truth. The fault must instead lie with its fallible human subjects. And so with each such question, with each advance of the power/knowledge dynamics of romantic discourse into her life, Petra is taken further and further away from other possibilities, becoming further entrenched in the social and experiential universe constructed by that discourse. In terms of discourses of romantic love, this is precisely what one must do in order to find the holy grail of happiness and fulfilment.

Naturalistic descriptions inevitably undermine the validity and visibility of alternative descriptions. It becomes a case of what is considered true versus what is false, as specified by the discourse in question (e.g., romantic love). Such a tactic puts the matter beyond dispute, making it possible to ignore or dismiss out of hand a range of other narratives or interpretive possibilities. Discourse conceals its status *as discourse*; as just one of a universe of ways of thinking and being in the world.

Discourses are intrinsically neither good nor bad

This is the final aspect of power/knowledge that I want to refer to. From a Foucauldian post-structural perspective, there can be no listing of 'good' versus 'bad' discourses. In a heavily criticized move (most notably by Habermas, 1990), Foucault refuses to make any normative pronouncements, because to do so would involve the valorization of certain ways of being in the world, and the devaluation of others.

For Foucault, any declaration of normative standards, by which to distinguish good discourses from worse ones, would amount to the assumption of a kind of governmental position relative to the issues being studied; as if one could adopt a God's-eye view of the social world and declare how things should work. Any elevation in truth or moral status of one kind of discourse (e.g., psychiatric or psychological knowledges) over another (e.g., local knowledges) would produce its own set of norms and unleash its own effects of power. Thus, Foucault is profoundly critical of anyone – a philosopher, a psychologist, a therapist – making a priori, universal, decontextualized judgements of right or wrong, of truth or falsehood, or even of how these things should be calculated. The traditional culturally valued methods of discernment, such as rationality, universal morality, or science, all of which offer methods to determine how things should be, cannot possibly take into account the specificity of each person's, and each community's, contexts, circumstances, and power relations. And so, instead of pretending he is able to stand in a position of supreme oversight, Foucault prefers – in what Habermas (1990) sees as a relativist position – to leave decisions of what is better or worse to the people and communities embroiled in their own discursive and power situations. It is in this sense that I understand narrative therapy's prioritization of each person's 'preferences' for living.

Neither, from this point of view, can we distinguish discourses on the basis of the presence or absence of power. Because 'power is everywhere' (Foucault, 1992, p. 93), inextricably tied up with human social interaction, it would be naïve to strive for anything like a power-free situation. 'Power is not evil', Foucault says elsewhere (1997d, p. 298). It is simply the case that a discourse without the support of power could have no effect in the world. It is interesting to note, in this respect, that at one point, postmodern therapists Anderson and Goolishian (e.g., 1990) sought to develop a therapy that removed power from the therapeutic relationship. They rejected 'the position that power and control are essential concepts either to the understanding or the practice of the therapeutic process' (p. 161). In converting therapy from what they described as a monological (power-infused) to a dialogical (non-power) endeavour, and in moving from a knowing to a 'not-knowing' stance, their intention was to make power and control 'nonproblems' in their practices (p. 160). Anderson and Goolishian have succeeded in highlighting a very important question: how can we avoid imposing our expert theories on our clients? But it is evident that not-knowing practices (like any other) retain significant, although obscured, power dynamics. For example, if we consider that power is not a one-way process, then it becomes clear that the client's positioning of *the therapist* would play a significant role in the power dynamics of that relationship. Furthermore, the discourse of 'not knowing' might have its own effects, such as frustrating a client who wants expert answers. And the removal of expert knowledges from the dialogue – the primary sense in which Anderson and Goolishian sought to render power a nonproblem – does not prevent a wide range of other kinds of knowledges (and hence power) from circulating in their practices. After all, no meaning can be constructed in the absence of knowledge practices.

The point is that power dynamics are unavoidable, particularly given that knowledge – power's omnipresent partner – is necessary for our being in the world. According to Foucault (1980b),

> there is no point in dreaming of a time when knowledge will cease to depend on power; this is just a way of reviving humanism in

a utopian guise. It is not possible for power to be exercised without knowledge, it is impossible for knowledge not to engender power. (p. 52)

We cannot divorce knowledge from power. The reader might be forgiven for thinking that I have been implicitly building an argument against discourses of romantic love. But I am not. As social analysts we might be critical of the effects of romantic discourse (as Burr has discussed it), but we should not imagine that there is some perfect, power-free discursive formation out there that we should find with and for our clients. The solution to the problems associated with a particular set of discursive practices (e.g., those of idealized romantic discourse) is not to be found in any finalized form in some equitable, power-free discourse. Instead, the priority shifts to the exploration of discursive *options*, and hence to the possibility of movement and change. This is what Foucault refers to as 'freedom' (e.g., 1982, p. 221): not finding the 'right' discourse, but finding an ability to move between different discursive possibilities. The problem arises when discourses come to seem uncontestable, and when other ways of thinking, feeling, being, and doing become invisible or are disqualified. This kind of hegemonic discursive arrangement – whether it be in the life of an individual or in the broader cultural sphere – amounts to a fixing of power dynamics, in which resistance, and hence democratic process more broadly, becomes impossible (Laclau and Mouffe, 2001).

One implication of this is that if we cannot use the contents of a discourse to decide, a priori, on its goodness, it can be useful to evaluate it in terms of its performance and function relative to other discourses in a particular historical era and set of cultural circumstances. A discourse which seems to fix power and close down alternative possibilities at one historical point might usefully break up precisely such hegemonic crystallizations of power at another point in time. For example, in the early twentieth century Freud's psychoanalytic discourse, even as it promoted its own power dynamics, represented a remarkably liberating alternative to such strategies as incarceration, social alienation, shock therapies, and lobotomies (c.f., Dreyfus and Rabinow, 1982). And yet, at a later point, narrative and other kinds of therapies arose, critiquing psychoanalysis in turn not only for its own limitations, but also for the hegemonic status it began to assume in mental health circles and even more broadly (as the example of homosexuality indicates). The problem with hegemonic achievement is, once again, the removal of diversity and the closing down of options; the silencing of a range of other voices, opinions, beliefs, and human practices. And so what is needed, from a post-structural perspective, is not an attempt to discover the correct, most truthful, most ethical, or most peaceful discourse, but the continual deconstruction and opening up of closed, hegemonic arrangements.

On this reasoning then, discourses of romantic love become problematic when a person is locked into them, and when there are no other options available for meaning-making; when these discourses assume hegemonic status. So when we note the powerful paralysing impact of discourses of romantic love on Petra's life, we should not imagine that we have discovered something intrinsically noxious – a malicious, strategically designed cover story for power – that should be exorcized from society, or from her life. Rather, from Petra we have heard about a discourse that is making it difficult for her to explore other options for finding meaning, fulfilment, and purpose. And, indeed, from Naffine (1994) and many others we have heard that this may apply to many more women than men. This discourse, right at this moment, has Petra – and many others – in its grip and is impeding her own capacity to move forward. If Petra cannot locate herself meaningfully, with some degree of thickness, in some other narrative then her constraint within the discourse of romantic love leaves her especially vulnerable to its effects when things go wrong. Thus, with the loss of her husband she suddenly experiences herself as having nowhere else to go, narratively speaking. She has only one visible life territory, and it is now barren. There is no-one else she can be, other than a failed romantic. It is such a fixing of the person in a particular discourse that can become problematic; not the contents of the discourse itself.

So who is the person in all of this?

This exploration of some of the key aspects of power/knowledge dynamics is intended to set the scene for a more focused discussion on the human being as a constituted subject. If power/knowledge refers to the forms and forces that act on persons, then what does the subject it constitutes look like? This is an important question, because it is precisely this constituted subject that we meet in our daily practices. That person is the 'product of power' (Foucault, 1983, p. xiv), and it is our acknowledgement of this that informs and underpins narrative therapy's constitutionalist perspective.

3
The Constituted Subject

In order to understand what it means to be a constituted subject, we must first be clear about what we have lost in our thinking: the true, essential, sovereign self that has occupied centre stage in psychology and psychotherapy for more than 100 years. There is, for us, no substantive, essential, core self. This point is repeatedly made in the works of both Foucault (e.g., 1966) and White (e.g., 2004), and is an implication of the constitutionalist power/knowledge formulation. There are no preexisting personality types, characteristics, or categories into which we normatively grow, and from which we might deviate into abnormality. When we experience personal difficulties, traumas, losses, conflicts, or anxieties, we should not imagine that we are thereby alienated from, or that we have lost touch with, the core of who we 'really are'. And when we overcome such difficulties, resolve our conflicts and ambivalences, recover from traumas or losses, we cannot reassure ourselves that there is some original, undamaged, authentic self to which we can return.

This is the first thing to be said about the human being from the perspective of narrative practice. As post-structurally oriented practitioners, we accept that there is no natural or universal human nature to ground our thought about the person (c.f., White, 1993). As Foucault (1988a) put it, 'I do indeed believe that there is no sovereign, founding subject, a universal form of subject to be found everywhere' (p. 50). This is, in fact, quite a significant loss in the context of our traditional habits of thought. It means, looking at the span of psychological discourse, that we cannot fall back on a grounding belief that, for instance, people are basically good, or genetically selfish, or inherently oriented towards personal growth. We cannot insist that at root, human beings have a natural growth tendency, search to become more 'themselves', or to realize their true potential, such as is thought in the humanistic tradition;

we cannot assume that people are innately driven to appraise their lives using rational methodologies, as some of our cognitive behavioural colleagues might argue; and we cannot assume, in the manner of classical psychoanalysis, that the essential drive of the human being is to balance out pleasure with the demands of reality. There are no such roots or essences lying at the heart of human experience.

Nevertheless, this notion of essences stubbornly refuses to go away. It easily creeps into our thinking, occasionally showing up, for instance, in our own talk about externalizing conversations. Our humanistic heritage seems to push us to imagine that the distance between 'persons' and 'problems' engendered via externalization frees us to see our 'clients as who they *are*' (Shulman, 1996, p. xii, emphasis added); as if there were some real, substantial, core person living behind or beneath the problem.

Still, we have in principle, if not always in practice, tried to rid ourselves of the illusion of the essential human being. It is not surprising then, that it is difficult for those of us working within the post-structural narrative tradition to answer the question of who the person is, in any positive, affirmative sense; in ways that our humanist, cognitive, or psychoanalytic colleagues have done. It is as if this is not the right question for us. Our theoretical question has not been: 'What is the self?' Rather, as the discussion in previous chapters suggests, if there is a question about the self at all, it must be something like: 'How, and into what, is the self produced?'

From this perspective, if the self is anything, it must be a product; not a thing that exists in itself, but a social, cultural, and historical product. This is what Foucault means when he tells us that the socially recognizable human being – the person I am, and the person with whom I interact (the 'you') – is not a 'substance' but a 'form' (Foucault, 1997d, p. 290). In Nietzschean terms, we can have a culture, but not a nature (Smith, 1996). As narrative practitioners, rather than searching for some 'substance' beneath the 'form', some nature beneath the culture, or a truth beneath the surface, we assume that the self *begins* with the meaning, the interpretation, the stories that give the person a particular shape or form. I suggest that, following Foucault, we are postmodern Nietzscheans, who believe that the self is always an interpretation, and that any search for the depths of this self will never lead to some atomistic centre to conveniently ground our interpretations. We will only find more interpretations. Lingis (1977) goes even further in his comment on this Nietzschean stance: 'Properly speaking, there are no longer ... any persons. There are ... only interpretations and interpretations of interpretations. There are no persons, selves, egos; there are only masks and masks of masks' (p. 42). The self is not a nodule of life which is crafted into a social product; it is rather the product itself.

As a social product, this self is always socially situated and invested with social meanings. It receives a place or places relative to other similarly produced selves, through which social activities can be coordinated. In other words, the form assigned a self is always an interpretation within more or less coordinated social networks of meaning. As Michael White (2004) tells us, in order to comprehend the individual's form – his or her 'personality', 'identity', or 'sense of self' – we must look not to the inside, to the intrapsychic or the psychological, but rather to the broader context of social conditions, knowledges, and practices that tell us what this body (e.g., male or female, black or white, young or old), and this conduct (e.g., masculine, feminine, mature, immature), can mean. As narrative practitioners we theorize that social practices and knowledges are carried onto our bodies, into our lives, represented in narrative form, and thereby constitute our identities.

But, as will have become clear in Chapter 1, there is a problem here: in contrast to the view of the person as a self-contained, self-determining being, which has predominated Western common-sense and psychological discourse (Sampson, 1993), does this vision of the socially produced self not represent the person in a docile, even pessimistic, way? What about free choice, intentions, personal agency? Are these too socially produced?

It is at this point that I believe we should resist the temptation into optimism that we so often find in narrative practice generally, and in Michael White's work in particular. I have argued that this poststructural account does indeed contain a degree of pessimism in its depiction of the person as a captured, obedient, and controlled body, especially when contrasted with the more widely accepted humanistic vision of the self as a self-determining figure, who can create his or her own meaning and life circumstances, unencumbered by societal power dynamics. Let us acknowledge it is not as easy as that, and that social forces frequently operate to make personal change difficult, and limit the kinds of changes one can even envision. This is not to promote a kind of social determinism. And Foucault strongly disavowed such an interpretation: 'The idea that power is a system of domination which controls everything and which leaves no room for freedom cannot be attributed to me' (1997d, p. 293). But at the same time we are not naïve optimists. I believe that a degree of pessimism, associated with a view of the socio-linguistically captured person, is justified to a far greater degree than is usually acknowledged in the narrative therapy literature (or even in discussions of Foucault's work). I do not want to rationalize away the docility or passivity implied in this vision of the person, but rather to explore how and why this matters from a therapeutic perspective.

We begin here with a discussion of the socially constituted subject, but I want to reiterate that we will not let matters stand there. Indeed, it is from the somewhat pessimistic platform of the socially constructed, sculpted human figure, that I hope, in the end, to generate a post-structural account of hope, personal agency, intentionality, and choice in the context of narrative practice.

Why must we be constituted subjects?

In order to understand what it means to be a constituted subject, let us consider the relationship between the person and knowledge or truth. As has already been made clear, our existence as subjects of knowledge is inevitably tied to, and shaped by, our interest in truth; in knowing. But why must we know ourselves, and end up as constituted subjects in the process? Foucault suggests that this interest – the will to truth – is socially constructed; a value that is a product of our time and context. Similarly, Dreyfus and Rabinow (1982), in their discussion of Foucault's work, see this desire to know the truth about ourselves as culturally produced (p. 174).

But it is interesting to consider Nietzsche's view that believing is more fundamental than that. In order to survive at all, he says, living beings must have 'a great deal of *belief*', and no 'doubt concerning all essential values... Therefore, what is needed', he goes on to say, 'is that something must be held to be true – *not* that something *is* true' (Nietzsche, 1968, p. 276). From this perspective, it is not only our society, and at only a particular point in history, that tells us we must know. It is essential to life itself. Any living thing, says Nietzsche, could not survive if it did not believe *something*, if it did not cling to some 'essential values' with absolute certainty.

Of course, our post-structural commitments – inspired by none other than Nietzsche himself (Deleuze, 2006; Hoy, 2004) – have us accepting that there is no final truth to be found. But how can one live this way – knowing that our truths are anything but – without collapsing into nihilism? For Nietzsche, we cannot. We must suspend this particular insight into the untruth of truth if we are to hold any commitments, values, positions, or principles at all. More to the point, if we do not believe in some truth we are at risk of being swept passively away in a sea of discourse; plunged into a world of fluid, unstructured, chaotic relativism.

Yes, we do want some fluidity in our identity options. This much is infused throughout much of the feminist, postmodern, post-structural, and narrative therapy literature. And to some extent this desire to emphasize the possibilities of fluidity may well be a product of, and a resistance against, the omnipresence of modern power and its thrust to produce us as something like self-contained individuals. Such resistance is surely a function of our current situation, and I support it, even as I here take the Nietzschean position that regardless of our cultural and historical circumstances, living beings need to believe *something*, to value something, to *be* something or somebody. The forces of constitution provide us with the *contents* of our beliefs and values. It is only as a constituted subject that we become somebody in particular. But for this to work we must simultaneously suspend our awareness that the form of self we assume is not essentially true. That is, we must, to all intents and purposes, believe that this is who we are, and forget that we know it is not. Nietzsche was not promoting an ironic or insincere self. And so in some respects we must become obedient converts to the discourses that claim us and give us meaning.

It follows from this argument that there is a problem with an existential, experiential, *lived* acceptance of a fully postmodern position, in which there is no final meaning, and that each person is, at root, nothing in particular. Nietzsche makes clear what Foucault did not: we cannot really live this way, with such a thoroughly relativistic perspective on ourselves and our lives. This would be to undermine meaning itself. Smith (1996) sees in Nietzsche the view that 'man is a nothing' and therefore needs 'discipline' – the imposition of order, structure, discourse – in order to forge a life (p. 149). I agree too with Stuart Hall (1985), who says that if we did not in some way fix or arrest the fluidity and infinite changeability suggested by postmodernism, we could have 'no...meaning at all!' (p. 93). Without beliefs, values, commitments, and a suspension of doubt about their truth, there could be no social order, and no sense of oneself as capable of engaging intentionally with that order. We need, in a sense, to adopt, internalize, or identify with one or other system of social constructs in order to *be* anything, or to say anything about ourselves.

So the Nietzschean position, adopted here, is that the need to hold something as true already lies 'within' us. So central is this compulsion to 'infer' truth that Nietzsche says not only that it is 'part of us', but that 'we almost *are* this instinct' (p. 278; I will take up this position further in Chapter 5). The systems, categories, and 'schemas' that develop in response to our need for truth are 'conditions of life for us' (Nietzsche, 1968, p. 278). Without them – as Heidegger interprets Nietzsche – we risk collapsing into 'dissolution and annihilation' (Heidegger, 1987, p. 85). On this account, then, the human being must search for meaning. But since he or she is 'a nothing' in particular, he or she cannot furnish its contents. It is on the question of where we find these truths that post-structural narrative versions of personhood depart from many modernist visions of the person. For the latter, the truth about one's 'self' is often presumed to lie hidden somewhere *within* the individual. As we have seen, for example, the psychoanalyst might locate this in the tensions between the instinctual pleasure principle and the ego's reality principle. But for the narrative practitioner, the truth about the self – the truth that Nietzsche tells us we need for life – does not emerge from within the person, but rather, following Foucault, originates in the social discourses in which we live our lives. As Wittgenstein might have put it, we are as immersed in these discourses as fish are in water (Segal, 1986).

The person relies on discourse to provide him or her with something substantial, some story, to believe in and value. He or she must therefore become a constituted subject. However, much of the time this does not entail freely selecting from among the complex range of discourses for a belief and set of values to identify with and adopt as his or her own (although we shall see in later chapters, such deliberate identification is indeed possible, especially as a means to subvert one's discursive constitution). There is no informed subject behind what Nietzsche sees as our inbuilt search for meaning. After all, the person relies on discourse for meaning, and is in no a priori position to assess various discourses for their suitability; such skills and know-how rely on the person already being well versed in discourse. The Nietzschean figure, then, must be receptive to being claimed by and becoming obedient to truth's requirements, but cannot make discernments about discourse until he or she is already a discursive subject – and hence, prejudiced in one way or another. Rather, things tend to work the other way round: it is discourse that selects and fashions the person. We have no choice but to comply, somewhere and somehow, because we thereby acquire what we need: a 'great deal of belief' and certain 'essential values', which grant us a place in the world and prevent our collapse into meaninglessness.

There is a significant implication of this line of reasoning: subjection is not inherently problematic. Rather, it is the very way in which we satisfy our need to believe in and value something, and hence to make meaning of our lives. But in our work we see every day that problems can and do emerge. Very often when people come to therapy they are not only 'strongly influenced by the overall cultural discourses in which they live on a day-to-day basis', as we all are, but are specifically 'caught in the grips of a dominant negative story' (Duvall and Beres, 2011, p. 34). Duvall and Beres are referring here to the person who is not only a constituted subject, but is constituted in a particularly problematic way. Perhaps the gripping story has the person positioned as stuck, paralysed, overwhelmed, confused, bewildered, or hopeless. This is a person constituted, or given shape, in so powerful a way that change might seem impossible.

What is the constituted subject?

So, let us agree that the constituted subject is the shape given to a person by the power/knowledge dynamics in which his or her life plays out, and which circulate throughout society. What does this mean? I have found it useful to think of the constituted subject in terms of the following six interrelated processes: first, the constituted subject is pressed into compliance with the terms of the constituting discourse; second, this figure is installed in a specific set of subject positions, which inform identity, and through which he or she comes to recognize himself or herself; third, the constituted person is a discursively decentred but phenomenologically centred subject; fourth, this subject becomes a living representative or agent of the discourse that gives him or her form; fifth, the person is a member of a community of subjection, which serves to sustain particular ways of knowing and doing, and thereby holds the person to his or her discursive position; and sixth, the person is a carrier of knowledges that have been downgraded or disqualified in the face of predominant constitutive discourses.

This is not intended to be a comprehensive list of the features of the constitutive subject. It is merely my way of making sense of the discursive shaping of the individual, which informs my understanding of the persons who come to talk to me about their problems in living. Let us now examine each of these processes in turn.

The constituted subject is pressed into compliance

As socially produced subjects of knowledge, we are pressed to comply with the dictates of those discourses which constitute us. Indeed, we often experience ourselves not as the agentive, intentional, fluid, and multiple agents that narrative and constructionist thinkers suggest we 'really' are, but in ways that suggest we have unwittingly identified with and become constrained within the discourses that circulate about us. We are sometimes constrained in our abilities to change our lives to such an extent that we seem more like passive 'social constructs' than 'autonomous agents' – which is how Bevir (1999, p. 67) describes the Foucauldian human being. While this description does not factor in the degree of personal agency built into the Nietzschean or Foucauldian visions of the person (as we shall see in later chapters), the idea that we are by-products of discourse reasonably reflects certain aspects of our lives; particularly when we become stuck in certain fixed identities or senses of self, whether they are problem-saturated or not. As such, to the extent that we are subjects of discourse, we become its service-able constructs, like cast members of a play whose lines and actions are pre-scripted. We become obedient.

Consider the case of Oscar, a friendly but dejected looking man, with a soft handshake and downcast eyes, who, at the age of 27, sought therapy for help with his suicidal thoughts and intense feelings of anxiety. This anxiety sometimes culminated in what he, following in the footsteps of his cultural practices, called 'panic attacks'. I asked Oscar what he thought these experiences were about, and he described a traumatic history of being beaten by his ex-partner, Alice, whom he had left three years prior to our first meeting. He told me how she had assaulted him on several occasions while they were together. Once she hit him on the head with a spanner and knocked him unconscious. When he came round he drove himself to the emergency room where he received stitches. We know, from research and clinical experience, that partner physical violence often involves multiple and complex emotional responses, including anger, shame, humiliation, and sometimes even a desire to protect the reputation of the person who perpetrated the abuse. Cognizant of these knowledges, I asked Oscar how he explained his injuries to the doctor and the nurses who stitched him up. He said that he decided not to divulge the truth of what had happened, but created some story to rationalize his injuries. I asked why he did this. He said it was not to protect Alice, but to protect himself from the humiliation of being seen as 'a weak man'. He felt that if the medical team knew what was really going on, he would not 'as a man', be able to 'look them in the eye'. He had absorbed what O'Leary (1999) describes as one of the most 'dominant constructions of manhood...Males are not supposed to be "victims"' (p. 164). In other words, Oscar found himself complying with certain requirements of acceptable masculine behaviour: tell a story that allows you to come across as 'a man', so you can 'look them in the eye'.

In this conversation, Oscar and I seemed to be moving towards a good sense of the expectations and ways of knowing that governed his behaviour; to which he had become obedient. I sought to clarify my understanding:

> I just want to see if I understand what was happening for you. You said you're a 'weak man'. Is it that you felt so ashamed that as a man you were being beaten by your partner, that you couldn't say this to anyone? It would be too shameful for them to know this about you?

He said this was exactly right, he was too ashamed.

I will return to this case below. For now, let us note Oscar's positioning in a cultural narrative of masculinity as a weak man; and as someone who is ashamed of this and seeks to hide it from others. In terms of our discussion, we see his obedience to the discursive requirement that a 'real man' should be a certain way, and present himself in certain ways to others. We gain the impression that these are ideas about masculinity and manhood that he has come to hold as final, unquestioned, even obvious truths. These truths incorporate what for Nietzsche might be considered 'essential values' (e.g., about masculinity), about which there is little room for doubt in Oscar's current experience and ways of knowing. It doesn't have to be true; but we have to believe in *something*, says Nietzsche. And in many communities, certain modes of masculinity have come to be valued as indicators of 'real men'. This forms a socio-culturally and historically horizon of meaning for Oscar. It is not that he is essentially a failure as a man, but rather he has inadvertently become obedient to particular requirements that in some senses he cannot fulfil; but which in another sense he fulfils very well. That is, on the one hand he cannot be the 'man' that he is expected to be. But on the other hand, his conduct – his experience of shame, his decision not to tell the doctors the real story, his desire to present himself as masculine and to look people in the eye – is precisely what one might expect of a man who values masculinity but feels he does not measure up. He must feel privately ashamed of himself, while publicly concealing his weakness. These concealing actions point to his continued compliance with the ideals of masculinity.

I use the words 'compliance' or 'obedience' here for a few reasons. These might seem unfair, even ungenerous terms to use, and certainly there are other reasonable and valid ways to characterize the person's relationship to discourse. Perhaps the person 'identifies' with or 'internalizes' a discourse; or he or she is 'recruited' into, 'governed' by, or 'positioned' within it. To some extent, all of these characterizations are useful, and the reader will notice that I use all of these terms from time to time. But each tells a slightly different story; and in each case, only part of the story. Of course, the terms I have chosen – compliance and obedience – also only offer a partial account, but I believe they are better starting points than other terms for understanding the processes of subjection.

The first advantage of the language of compliance is that it points our gaze in a particular direction. It pushes us to ask: if we are complying, what is it that we are complying with? The primary author of our self-understandings, in other words, is not ourselves, but those forces with which we tend to comply; those forces which seek to govern our lives and our identities. This term creates an image of external rules, requirements, standards, and expectations that precede us, and which do not begin their lives 'inside' us. Instead, they come from the outside, swarming into our lives from all directions. Consider the hold that discourses of masculinity, femininity, success, and work ethic can exert over our lives, activities, and sense of self-worth: these discourses promote standards and expectations that we, as individuals, did not create, but which we find almost impossible to ignore. Indeed, they easily form the horizons of our meaning-making capacities, such that they block our vision of other possibilities (Veyne, 2010). What is the alternative to success? Well, failure of course!

While the language of compliance directs our gaze to the outside, it nevertheless remains difficult to identify the agents of these requirements. This can be a source of confusion in some narrative thought. I think it is a mistake to imagine, as Freedman and Combs (1996) suggest, that particular persons or organizations 'control the discourses of power in our culture', and 'gaze' down on the rest of us (p. 39). Once again, we have reason to wonder if the Marxist discourse of the powerful few exploiting the dominated masses continues to affect our thinking on issues of power. Rather, in the Foucauldian view the author of selves and of lives is all but invisible, and retains an elusive, vague, even insubstantial quality. The forces which command us – or persuade, cajole, influence us – do not conveniently originate in some single authoritarian source: an oppressive father, a bullying boss, the ruling classes, or the government. These figures might be relay points for power, and they may well have been recruited as representatives of its discourses, but they too are obedient subjects, albeit differently positioned.

One way of thinking about the agent enforcing our compliance is via what Veyne (2010), through his translator, calls the 'set-up' (p. 9; another term for Foucault's word 'dispositif'): the institutionally and socially coordinated activities that sustain particular ways of doing and thinking. The fact that power operates through a more or less coordinated network of persons and practices leads to the sense that these constitutive forces – as we shall see in the case of Oscar – come 'from *everywhere*' (Foucault, 1990a, p. 93, emphasis added): movies, novels, advertisements, countless other media, common-sense discourse, and even from well-meaning friends and family.

While Nietzsche says we must believe something, without any doubts, Foucault shows us that there is at the same time a kind of socio-historical law at work: the believed something must remain within the horizons of meaning set by our sociocultural and historical situations. We must find our truth within this boundaried set of practices and knowledges if we are to be recognized as valid social partners and appropriate social actors. We have seen that Oscar's shame and concealment point to such compliance, insofar as these experiences allow him to remain recognizable as a man within the discursive framework of masculinity. Likewise, Petra's distress in the face of the failure of her romance (see Chapter 2) may reveal a degree of compliance with the requirement that women should identify themselves solely in and through their romantic attachments (c.f., Naffine, 1994). A total collapse not only of hope, but also of a sense of self, is in keeping with the failure of such a vital, identity-giving, relationship. The notion of compliance – unlike the idea of 'identification', for instance – points our interpretive gaze outwards towards such requirements.

The second advantage of the term 'compliance' is, perhaps paradoxically, that it assumes a level of agency on the part of the person. It posits a two-way relationship, between discursive prescriptions and the subject who either complies with them or does not. On the one hand, the notions of 'identifying with' or 'becoming attached to' certain sociocultural expectations also convey a sense of agency, but perhaps too much. They do not sufficiently highlight the degree to which we are subjected to – we tend not to choose – discursive requirements. On the other hand, Foucauldian discourse frequently and usefully deploys the notion of 'governance' to characterize the constituted subject's position relative to societal discourse and power dynamics (e.g., Foucault, 1982; and I will also use the term), but I think the idea of being governed minimizes our view of the person's agency. Governance is something done to a person. This is in some ways true of how we are positioned relative to discourse, but it obscures from view the person's response, which might take the form of either compliance or non-compliance. And this recognition of the person's response to discursive dictates brings us closer to an appreciation of his or her agency. In contrast to the idea of being governed, compliance is something a person *does*. It is an action, and in some respects, even an agentive action. Indeed, Foucault spoke often of the subjection of 'free subjects' (1982, p. 221), in the sense that we *can* disobey the requirements of discourse.

The problem with power, however, is that while obedience is supported, disobedience tends to be costly. For example, Oscar might decide to speak out against his abuse at the hands of his ex-partner, but in the context of a macho, masculinist culture, this may well lead to his being ridiculed for being beaten by a woman (as we shall see below). Similarly, Petra might one day protest against the unfair effects of romance, but this could trigger disapproval from her traditional parents, and leave her feeling lost, and like an outsider, relative to much of her romance-supporting social context.

These costs notwithstanding (and of course, re-authoring and other narrative practices can function to lend meaning to such resisting activity), the notion of compliance as action promotes the possibility of resistance against those subtle but almost omnipresent forces which impose unwanted identities (or social constructs) on the person. Resistance is clearly an important aspect of our thought. The thrust of Foucault's work in identifying prevailing discourses is not to enable our 'identification' with them, or our 'construction' or 'positioning' in their terms, but precisely to trouble them; to re-infuse the discursive field with dynamism, rather than allow it to drift towards closure and finality. It is fortunate, then, that the relationship between person and discourse is always a troubled one. Thinking about our position relative to discourse in terms of compliance invites us to think about resistance in a way that some other terms might not. In what might well be considered White and Epston's seminal case (1990, see pages 43–48), of a young boy with encopresis, six-year-old Nick and his family were, without realizing it, operating within the horizons of possibility set by Sneaky Poo – that is, they were complying with its requirements – before finding ways to unsettle that relation of obedience. The notion of compliance serves to bring the troubled relationship between person and discourse into sharp relief.

To be clear, compliance is not a feature of only the most distressed, stuck, or impotent clients. We are all to some extent obedient to the social order (via its discourses and practices) for most of our lives, and in most of our activities. For example, we must observe cultural expectations of language use in order to be understood. Even now as I write, I am surely adhering to at least some set of norms and expectations concerning academic and therapeutic writing. Similarly, in order to relate meaningfully to our social partners, we must share understandings and performances of culturally salient domains such as gender, justice, emotion, and even problems of living, such as depression, sadness, anxiety, and so on: the kinds of things that matter to many communities at this point in our histories. We would be considered alien, and beyond the pale of social recognizability, if we did not orient our actions and senses of self in some way to such culturally shared ways of knowing; if we did not, in more or less socially coordinated fashion, pin ourselves to certain shared elements of meaning. A level of discursive compliance, which entails holding up as true and natural, and acting in accordance with, certain cultural knowledges and expectations, is necessary for meaningful social engagement and self-understanding. But clearly this does not mean it is always advantageous.

Externalization is a useful narrative response to unwitting compliance, as White and Epston (e.g., 1990) have demonstrated on countless occasions. Thus, our externalizing thoughts turn to the prescriptions, expectations, and requirements of these discourses; the expectations to which Oscar and others have become obedient. In turn, this enables resistance to be directed at those discourses.

I want to make the point that I use the terms compliance and obedience here in a conceptual rather than pragmatic way. In practice, when talking with people in distress, one might not necessarily use such provocative terms to characterize a person's relationship to the discursive expectations that operate so powerfully in his or her life. Other metaphors that might come up in dialogue include the idea of being persuaded or cajoled, being told what to do, being dictated to, being seduced into thinking this or that, being issued with requirements, being conscripted into expectations or rules, and so on (see White, 2007). For example, I did not say to Oscar, 'It seems you have become obedient to the requirements of masculinity', but rather, 'It sounds to me like you've bought into certain expectations about how a man should be'. But I find it useful as a therapist to think of how the person complies, so that I can more starkly perceive how she or he resists.

A positioned subject

The capacity of discourse to produce social realities in its own terms is dependent on its ability to produce human subjects of specific types, shapes, or forms. When Foucault defines discourses as 'practices that systematically form the objects of which they speak' (p. 49), we should remember that we are among those objects. Discourses speak of us in particular ways, and to the extent that they are deployed in various socially aligned activities, we are pressed to become what they say we are. For example, and while real life is more dynamic and more complex than this, we can agree in principle that a psychiatric discourse requires such figures as doctors and patients, just as discourses of masculinity need macho men, weakling men, fawning women, emasculating women, and discourses of romantic love need right persons and soul mates, wrong persons and betrayers, and so on. For such practices to be realized in the social world, people must be shaped into the mutually appropriate forms. We must play our parts to bring the terms of discourse into existence. We cannot avoid discourse, and so our only means for making sense of who we are is to situate ourselves – or be situated – in some or other of the positions they provide.

I find it useful to think of these discursively produced forms, such as Petra's sense of herself as 'a hopeless romantic' and Oscar's idea of himself as 'a weak man', through the notion of 'subject positions' (see Torronen, 2001, for a useful discussion on various uses of this term); a concept which is being used explicitly by some in narrative practice (e.g., Bird, 2004; Winslade, 2005). While we noted above that the person is pressed to comply with the requirements of discourse, the notion of the subject position refers to the specific contents of those prescriptions: the 'character slots', or specific forms, assigned to people by the particular narratives in which they live. Discourses align our social activities by shaping us into all manner of historically specific, socially recognizable, and culturally relevant forms: competent professionals, kind parents, strict teachers, jealous husbands, black sheep, sexual deviants, hopeless romantics, weak men, and so on. In an important sense, we become who we are by finding and recognizing ourselves – our positions – in socially available discourse. This is what is meant by the phrase, commonly used in narrative therapy, that stories 'are directly constitutive of life' (White, 1993, p. 125) and of identity (Freedman and Combs, 1996).

More technically, Torronen (2001) defines the subject position as

> a construction which, on the one hand, evolves in a specific relation to the audience and to the existing subject positions in a particular context of interaction and which, on the other hand, obtains its meaning by being attached situationally to categories and story lines. (320)

Here, we see that the assignment and inhabitation of subject positions gives the person a meaningful place in at least two respects: a narrative position, and a social position.

First, the person occupies a place within the narrative itself, in relation to the story's 'categories and story lines'. This place allows enculturated others – others who have been recruited into playing the same kinds of cultural games – and the person himself or herself, to 'understand' something about the person. His or her conduct and experience is given a kind of socially and personally recognizable sensibility. For instance, the psychiatric patient might be positioned as 'crazy' within particular narratives, and it is expected that enculturated persons would recognize the sense – the meaning – of this.

But subject positioning could not be sustained without an active social network that reproduces the discourses and norms which hold us to a certain position. And so, second, the positioned person derives a place relative to others who participate directly or indirectly in that narrative's performance: the discourse's interpellated or subjectified community. These others are the 'audience' to which Torronen refers, although we should not be misled by that term into thinking of them as merely witnesses to the person's positioning. Rather, they are the person's discursive partners, also positioned with respect to the overarching discourse, and each of whom relates in some way to the person's, and each other's, subject positioning. Such a network of positions enables mutually coordinated activity, whose alignment as we saw in Chapter 2, makes up the primary force of power. For instance, psychiatric discourse might assign the patient certain personal positions ('schizophrenic', 'resistant'), which stand in specific relation to certain others, such as doctors, nurses, concerned family members, other patients, insurance companies, the law, and so on. This linked-up group of persons – or rather, positions – maintain, albeit invisibly, their own and each other's positions through their ongoing activities, and in turn reproduce psychiatric discourse and practice itself.

This second aspect of the positioning process is a vital aspect of the functioning of power/knowledge in our lives. Not only are we assigned positions in terms of sense or meaning, but also these meanings are socially enforced and upheld by our discursive, power/knowledge partners. These other persons – by virtue of their recognition of us, and our recognition of them – often help maintain us in our obedience, and hold us to our positions.

Let us recall, with respect to these two forms of positioning (the narrative and the social), Oscar's struggle in relation to himself as a weak man.

In our second session, he told me about his attempt to move away from this view of himself. He moved in with his father for a period of time after leaving Alice, and decided after years of silence to confide in him about his experiences and the shame he had suffered. Oscar was relieved to experience his father as sympathetic rather than judgemental, and he felt regret that he had not expressed his concerns before. He said he started to feel good again. Here, we see Oscar moving towards some alternative position; something other than masculine failure, and not quite masculine strength either. In other words, in these actions he is no longer complying with the requirements of masculine discourse (e.g., conceal your weakness, and feel private shame). Instead, he speaks about his situation rather than concealing it, and instead of shame, begins to feel he is doing something right. This act has the potential to represent a slight opening towards a new set of discourses, narratives, and self-positions. Might a new horizon of meaning, one that is not dominated by hegemonic discourses and practices of masculinity, open up through Oscar's engagements with his father? Indeed, Oscar initially began to feel empowered and hopeful, and felt that perhaps he no longer needed to hide in shame. He told me that he experienced 'the world opening up' in front of him.

But one evening a few days later this movement was undone when, after having a few drinks, Oscar's father, staring bleary eyed at him, asked: 'Tell me Oscar, how does a man allow that to happen? How can a woman beat up a man? How can a man allow his woman to beat him around like that?' Oscar was taken aback by his father's challenge, and told him that he just did not understand. Oscar left the house in tears. This confrontation was a devastating experience for him, and served to effectively pull him squarely back into the position of masculine failure from which he had been slowly edging away. The new world that he described as 'opening up' before him simply dissolved.

There are many features of this situation which we could look at more closely. But at this point I want to stress, with respect to the above discussion, that Oscar's positioning as a failure of a man entails both narrative and social positioning. First, with respect to his narrative positioning: his feeling that he is a 'failure' and 'a weak man' is inevitably grounded in broader narratives that make sense of, and give meaning to, these experiences. In this case, we are referred to broader cultural narratives and practices of masculinity and manhood, which provide a meaning-sense of his position. It is in relation to these that Oscar feels a failure, weak, humiliated, beaten, and vulnerable. This is how he is *supposed* to feel under these circumstances, in terms of the logic of this discourse, and thus his experience entails a kind of discursive compliance. This carries the important implication that Oscar is not under the influence of some kind of cognitive distortion or error in thinking. The notion of subject positioning highlights instead that Oscar's twin expectations – that being beaten by a woman is evidence of his weakness, and that people would publicly or privately judge him for this – are in some ways prescribed for him. To the extent that his social partners buy into and perform (i.e., comply with) these constructions, as his father did, they become 'true', and socially real. Indeed, he is *right* to hold these expectations, to the extent that they flow from the narrative logic of the overarching masculine discourse that has him in its grip. This is what his actions mean in a particular narrative and social space. His shameful response is, therefore, not just understandable but prescribed, appropriate, accurate, and rational. As we shall see in Chapter 6, understanding the person's responses in this way can be enormously beneficial when we are engaged in therapeutic dialogue.

Second, this positioning has a significant social element, in the sense that it locates Oscar in specific sorts of relationships with those around him. Indeed, his social partners are able to hold him to his assigned position, thereby revealing the recapturing power of social alignment: its capacity to bring the straying individual back into the discursive fold. Oscar's hesitant attempts to move away from the capturing discourse, and its problem-saturated positioning of him, were undone by his father's critical comments, effectively reminding him: this is not a matter of speaking out, a potentially new story, with new positioning possibilities; it is a matter of being a weak and ineffectual man. A whole social universe is produced as part of his recruitment into this position. For example, there is the powerful woman defeating the male weakling. There are various implicitly constructed others, such as those men who, we are led to believe, would not allow such a situation to have emerged in the first place (the 'normal' or 'strong' ones), and those who would (the 'weak' ones). There are other social participants, such as Oscar's father, who note the situation with disapproval and judgement. And then there is an entire population of virtual and less involved observers, such as the nurses and doctors who stitched him up in the hospital, who as enculturated persons stand at the ready, on the margins of Oscar's experience, waiting to pass judgement on him. It is reasonable to try and hide the truth from this ensemble of social actors, as Oscar did, because they, as fellow participants in the games of masculinity, are potential critics and enforcers of those games.

To the extent that we can say anything at all about ourselves as individuals, we have become subject to some discourse or other; we thereby inhabit subject positions. And insofar as knowledge cannot be separated from social power relations, each of us becomes 'a product of power' (Foucault, 1983, p. xiv), a 'variable of the statement' (Deleuze, 1988, p. 49), an 'effect' of or a 'position' in discourse (Hall, p. 23); even a 'social construct' (Bevir, 1999, p. 67). We become the kinds of people that discourse tells us we are.

However, as narrative therapists well know, persons are always multi-storied. In terms of the present discussion, this means that we are always multiply positioned in multiple societal discourses. This multiplicity allows for some degree of dynamic movement around the person's dominant, problem-saturated positions. Thus, Oscar is not only a failed man, despite his powerful sense of himself this way. He is also many other things: a 'computer genius', as a friend of his told him; a loving son to his parents; a caring brother to his sick sister, who was also caught up in a physically and emotionally abusive relationship; and so on. His sense of masculine failure has not been so successful that it totally centres his life or identity. He is, in this sense, ultimately a decentred rather than a centred subject. As therapists, these notions of multiplicity and decentredness give us hope. But we should remember that this hope does not match Oscar's feelings of hopelessness.

A discursively decentred, but phenomenologically centred subject

As post-structural thinkers, we cannot see the human being as a centred subject; a being who 'is' something in an essential, absolute, totalized, and unequivocal sense. Instead, we emphasize a vision of the person as discursively decentred. I will attempt here to distinguish between these notions of the centred and decentred subject.

The notion of centredness is well represented, if not always explicitly, in much therapeutic and common-sense talk. It is evoked in the use of such widely used phrases as 'it touches me to the core', 'try to centre yourself', or 'become who you really are'. Theoretically speaking, the centred figure is seen to comprise internal processes (which may be referred to as 'psychological' or 'emotional') organized by a singular set of principles, forces, or dynamics. These core dynamics, thought to lie at the heart of personal experience, are often presumed to suffer distortion or concealment in the face of troublesome life events. The task of 'finding oneself' – the singular truth of oneself – is therefore seen as a challenging task, for which psychotherapy is often recommended.

The notion of a centred self does not rule out multiplicity in action or in identity. But such diversity is treated in a reductionist manner, and often with suspicion rather than celebration. For the centred self, there cannot be several legitimate truths living alongside one another; there can be only one truth with many offspring, each bearing the mark of its parent.

But in the post-structural tradition, we want to reorient to this image of the centred being in two ways. First, we externalize rather than internalize the 'thing' that supposedly stands at the centre. And second, we notice that this externalized thing is not the only thing there. We recognize, in other words, that any subject position, or any sense of self, is but one of a multiplicity of positions and options for living. And we do so without collapsing this multiplicity into a singular truth. So we tend to notice the decentredness, multiplicity, and multi-voicedness of life, and thereby undermine any notion of life in terms of centredness, singularity, and single-voicedness. Let us consider each of these points.

First, on externalizing what is theoretically centred, I think it is important to clarify our picture of this process. The way I think about the notion of the centred being is to imagine this mythical figure, and his or her actions, not as animated by some internal core process (e.g., the intra-psychic tensions between ego and id), but by his or her obedience to some external principle, value, law or belief. That is, a centred being – if there can be such a thing – is one who is utterly and completely obedient to the requirements of the subject position he or she is assigned. This externalized image derives from the work of neo-Marxist philosopher Louis Althusser (1971/2008), who helped us shift from thinking of who we are in terms of *internal* places and mechanisms, to thinking of our positions and senses of self in terms of identifications with *external* ideas, values, principles, and so on, which serve as nodal points or fulcrums for particular social discourses and practices. These principles do not originate in us, but exist out there in the social world.

Thus, in order to make sense of the decentred subject, the first thing I recommend we do is change how we think about centredness: not in terms of the heart of the human psyche, but in terms of a social-discursive principle which attempts to stand at the centre of lived experience. Theoretically speaking then – and centredness can only exist in theory – a centred being can be thought of as one who identifies with, is obedient to, or governed by, just one such discursive centre. Althusser uses the term 'interpellation' to describe the manner of our recruitment into discourse. He noted that when we recognize ourselves in the calls that are made to us ('You're an anxious person!', says Tholani's mother;

'Yes, that's me!', replies Tholani), we are thereby interpellated or hailed into a subject position that stands as an anchor for particular discourses and practices (e.g., in the case of anxiety, the psy discourses and their ways of knowing and doing). To take this further, we could hypothesize, for instance, that what strives to be centred in Tholani's experience is a prescriptive vision of 'normality'; in Oscar's life, a certain principle of masculinity; in Petra's case, the culturally valued figure of the romantically attached woman; and so on. These are the principles that bind social participants together and orchestrate their activities such that the discourse itself is maintained and enhanced. We are led to think not in terms of who the person 'is', but in terms of what he or she has become by virtue of his or her compliance with some societal law or prescription.

Althusser's vision can be contrasted with the humanist tradition that continues to influence thought, in the Western world in particular, which invites us to think of ourselves in internalized terms; as if we possess these qualities (masculinity, romance, anxiousness) at the heart, at the centre, of our psyches. It is, as we shall discuss below, the preponderance of such an internalized view, via what Epston (1993) refers to as 'internalized discourses' (p. 161), that leads people in modern societies often to form negative identity conclusions, effectively conflating the external principles that have caught them in their orbit, with those persons' internal senses of who they are. Such internalizing accounts look in the wrong places; they mislocate the 'cores' and 'essences' of which they speak.

From a Foucauldian perspective, we would say that discourse is not so much concerned to hold the intra-psychic centre of the person in place, but rather to maintain its own principles *at the centre of social activity* (although some psychoanalytic colleagues might argue that this amounts to the same thing, via the psychic internalization and centring of an external law). Indeed, Laclau and Mouffe (2001) argue, in a manner aligned with Foucault, that one of the primary objectives of discourse is precisely to establish its own fixed centres – knowledges, principles, but also human figures (consider the Pope in Catholicism). By way of illustration, we can draw on Althusser's (1971/2008) use of the principle of God as the centre of Christian belief and practices. The idea here is that God does not live 'in' us, in the way that many Christian doctrines maintain, but rather that the *principle* of God moves around us, in the broader culture, inciting us to follow it, to orchestrate our activities around it, and to distance ourselves from other principles (e.g., other religious beliefs or practices). It strives thereby to be at the centre of social practice. The same can be said of the aggressive advances of masculinity (as we saw with Oscar) and romance (Petra) into the sociocultural network. This centring move is always a power move. It is part of a social power game, insofar as a pervasive discourse (e.g., masculinity, romance, or Christianity) is engaged in an ongoing tussle with other discourses, endeavouring to locate its own principles or ideas at the centre of human activity, and to displace – or perhaps neutralize, adapt, and incorporate – others; to have us move and dance around these principles, and not others. We can think of the achievement of such centredness in terms of 'hegemony' (Laclau and Mouffe, 2001, p. 7), or 'domination' (Foucault, 1997d, p. 283), in which power dynamics cease to be *dynamic*, resistance becomes impossible, and a single-voiced life is installed. It is fortunate then, that while this notion of centredness – conceived now externally, politically – serves a useful theoretical function, it is rarely if ever fully achieved in the empirical world.

And this is the second problem with the centredness thesis: discourse never captures us so completely that it stands alone at the centre of our experience. Laclau and Mouffe, as well as Foucault, largely attribute this relative failure of discourse to the inevitable multiplicity of discourse in the social arena. These authors move beyond Althusser's centred vision of social relations and dynamics to show that humans are always multiply positioned (this multiplicity does not feature in Althusser's work). Indeed, for the Foucauldian as well as the narrative practitioner, the existence of multiple discourses, stories, ways of being, and ways of thinking, tells us immediately that there can be no fully centred discourse. Other discourses are always competing to be represented as ways of thinking and doing. God – the principle, or nodal point – might centre Christianity, but there is always the tug of alternative religions and other ways of being in the world, which decentre this principle as a way of organizing the entire society's experiences and practices. This dynamic interplay between discourses effectively decentres the principle seeking centralization.

In sum, we can think of centredness in terms of internalization and reductive singularity, and decentredness in terms of externalization and multiplicity. And, since we are committed to a decentred ontology, we think of the principle to which the person has become obedient as existing out there in the social domain (Heller, 1996), and we recognize that there are always multiple principles competing to capture his or her actions, thoughts, emotions, and identity. This means that the decentred subject is always fragmented, or split, between multiple discourses (Foucault, 1972).

Nevertheless, as constituted subjects we often *experience* ourselves rather differently. Many of our experiences do not seem external and multiple, but internal and singular. Our decentred situation is often invisible, and therefore the tremendous advantages it affords are frequently unusable. Given the widespread humanist requirement that we know ourselves, and establish some form of stable identity, there is a tendency for persons to often *experience* themselves as centred, in either desirable or undesirable ways. Foucault's emphasis on the fragmentation of identity by discourse dynamics does not prevent him from recognizing that sometimes we have a unified self-experience. After all, some degree of unification allows us to be recognizable as this or that, over time, to ourselves and to others (Huijer, 1999). Thus, the person who describes acting from the 'core' of his or her being experiences a sense of utter personal congruence and flow; just as the person constituted in problem-saturated ways experiences these problems as central to his or her existence. So we might be discursively decentred subjects, but we are sometimes *phenomenologically* centred. This describes, I think, the situation of the constituted subject: decentred in the sense that he or she is never fully constituted as one particular type of subject, but centred in the sense that (1) these external principles feel internal, and (2) the range of alternative forms of subjection or identification do not seem 'real', or seem to have no noticeable impact on his or her life.

For example, Oscar recognizes himself in the sociocultural interpellative calls of masculinity, and so he understands that they refer to him as a self-contained, psychological being. Consequently, his masculine failures seem to point to his 'character' or 'personality'. We know as narrative observers that other subject positions are available to him, and that in certain moments he even adopts some of these (e.g., as a computer genius or a caring son). But his phenomenological experience of centredness limits the gravitas, and the impact, of such ways of thinking about and conducting himself. Unlike his constituted subjectivity which feels 'in here', these other options seem to be 'out there'; fantasies which cannot feel as real as the truths that he believes live in his soul. And so his self-assessments, or at least those which matter most to him and which feel the most true, come back in centripetal fashion to the issues of masculinity: that external discourse posing as an internal quality, and which from that place seems to tell the truth about who he really is. His life experience is thereby internalized, and its richness reduced to a singular theme.

A discursive representative

The fourth feature of the constituted subject is this: the person's seemingly centred position provides him or her with a perspective from which to engage with the world. The subject position can be thought of as an interpretive (and hence political/strategic) vantage point, colouring the world in discursively prescribed ways. And it is frequently from this vantage point that the person engages with the world. In this way, the person becomes a re-circulator of the discourse in question, a discursive agent, or representative, serving to spread the rationalities, values, and practices of that discourse.

The distinction between the person as discursive subject and discursive representative should not be made too sharply, because of course they are linked: it is through the person's position (e.g., as a romantic subject), and his or her identification with it, that he or she is able to represent to others, and to recruit others into, the values, norms, and practices of that particular discourse. Nevertheless, there are some important differences between the two. At a theoretical level, Foucault (1980c) makes a distinction between the subject as product and vehicle of power. That is, on the one hand the subject position is a place prescribed by discourse and enforced by power, the place into which the person is recruited. But from this place, and on the other hand, the person also becomes a recruiting agent, equipped to interpellate or subjectify others in particular ways. The person is therefore more than power's product; he or she is also its active 'relay point' (Weberman, 2000, p. 260), its 'dense point of transfer' (Foucault, 1990b, p. 103).

The person's ability to serve as a relay point for power can play out in any number of domains, including in the therapeutic relationship itself (Winslade, Crocket, and Monk, 1997). In my work with Oscar, for example, it was apparent that he effectively recruited me into the masculine ways of being that had come to matter to him. I sensed that I was being positioned as the kind of man he wanted to be, someone who was (in his eyes) successful, strong, and capable. In our sessions, I developed a dimly perceived sense of myself as this kind of figure in relation to his 'weak man' position. I became aware of my own sense of masculinity in our interactions, which was associated with my speaking a little more loudly and in a more forthright manner than I normally would. And in the manner of an older brother, I felt an urge to guide him and sometimes even to dismiss him. These are unusual responses for me in the context of my own work. It took me some time to recognize these feelings and the ways in which I had inadvertently inhabited the construct of the 'stronger man' made open by the discourse of masculinity to which he had become attached, and relayed into the room.

We will return to this episode later on, but for now I want to highlight that far from being the danger that Winslade and colleagues (1997) suggest such a positioning of the therapist by the client can be, my eventual recognition of what was happening ended up being very useful. I became aware that as a multiply constituted being, this was surely not the only way in which Oscar was positioning me; he would surely also interact with me in other ways too. Thus, it became possible to identify relational unique outcomes; ways in which he subtly undermined my 'authority' and removed me from my perch of superiority. I will take this up further in Chapter 6.

The notion of the person as a representative of the discourse that constitutes him or her reveals a certain paradox. As the person is recruited to be the docile, obedient subject of discourse, he or she becomes a political actor: a side-taking, biased, believing, faithful agent of particular power arrangements. The constituted subject can in principle never be a neutral observer or impartial participant in the world. Instead, the subject of power is transformed into its vehicle, transporting certain ways of knowing and doing into a host of interpersonal situations. In some ways at least, the person is always positioned on one side or other of some broader power struggle. For example, Oscar's investment in masculinity helps to support and recirculate a particular way of being a gendered figure, thereby unwittingly standing in opposition to ideas, beliefs, and values associated with other ways of being. Our obedience has us taking sides.

A participant in communities of subjection

Narrative therapists have used the notion of communities of concern (Freedman and Combs, 1996; Madigan and Epston, 1995) to refer to a grouping of people who participate in, or are members of, one's 'club of life' (White, 1997, p. 22). This community, made up of any number of individuals who are linked to the person, has proven to be extremely useful in supporting preferred developments in that person's life. White noticed that such a community could help thicken and socially legitimize the client's preferred identity narratives or ways of being, and so he would sometimes recruit them as witnesses to developments in the client's life.

While White's focus, to put the matter more formally, fell on the utilization of communities to facilitate the ongoing constitution and reconstitution of preferred subject positions, it is clearly the case that communities can support any number of social practices; whether they are preferred or not. We are inevitably members of what Madigan (2011) refers to as 'communities of discourse' (p. 49). What Madigan recognizes here is that it is discourse that organizes and gives shape to communities in the first place, recruiting diverse persons to serve some shared objective (the discursive centre, if you like), through the lure of certain ideas, promises, values, and rationales. A rugby or football team, a mental health team or organization, a couple, a family, a book club, a group of teens gathered on the street corner, a nation: all are discursively constituted communities to the extent that their activities are loosely, even if only transiently, orchestrated around some shared value, belief, or practice objective. The community functions in the form of power as we have already described: members loosely align their activities in such a way that compliance (with certain implicit or explicit objectives or values) is supported, while resistance is not.

Clearly, communities not only support preferred initiatives and personal projects, but can also serve to maintain us in our stuckness or our pain. Indeed, it is hard to imagine maintaining some degree of emotional distress, or a negative identity conclusion, without some loosely coordinated community supporting, rationalizing, or otherwise maintaining the values, stories, or positions associated with that distress. And so I propose that the person who seeks our assistance can be thought of as already part of a broader community of subjection; a community of people whose conduct sustains his or her problem-saturated positioning. It is perhaps clear by now that such communities do not necessarily resemble communities in the way we ordinarily use the term (e.g., a school community, or a neighbourhood community). The community of subjection might not have its own club-house, and its members might not even know each other. Those persons who unwittingly work together to hold us in our distress might include professionals, novelists and newsreaders, movie heroes, characters in television advertisements, as well as acquaintances, loved ones, friends, spouses, and family members. In these persons' diverse behaviours lie certain key activities which function in more or less (though not always intentionally) coordinated fashion to hold us to a particular kind of subject position. We saw in Chapter 2 that it is precisely this kind of socially aligned behaviour that Rouse (1994) and Wartenburg (1990) see as central to understanding what Foucault means by power.

Well-meaning and loving others can make up a community of subjection, as was evident in the experience of 15-year-old Nobisa. She came in with her parents and 13-year-old sister to meet with me, after it was discovered that she was pregnant. Her father, a church minis-ter, proclaimed the value of 'morality', 'chastity', and 'good, Christian morals'. He described them as a 'Christian family', for whom news of Nobisa's pregnancy came as 'a great and disappointing shock'. It was a shock too, Nobisa's mother told me, to the broader church community for whom this particular family's behaviour was always in the spotlight. She said this pregnancy threatened to undermine the family's credibility in the community, given her husband's prominent position. It seemed that a powerful community of subjection was ready to pass judgement on Nobisa, and on her family. When I asked Nobisa how she felt hear-ing all this, she looked at her mother for what I expected was support. Her mother told her to answer me. Nobisa said that she felt 'ashamed'. I asked what she was ashamed of, and she said people would see her as 'loose and immoral'. When I asked which people she had in mind, she simply said that she had let down her family and she was very sorry. I guessed that she was overwhelmed and exhausted at having to explain herself, and at being the focus of all this judgement.

It was evident that Nobisa felt negatively judged from all angles; as we have already seen, power seems to come from everywhere (Foucault, 1990a), labouring in multiple and diverse ways to shape the person's conduct such that it conforms to the dictates of particular discourses. In this discourse of Christian moral responsibility, supported by a wide network of people, Nobisa was assigned a position of shame. Although she did not believe herself that she was 'immoral' or 'loose', she did state her belief that she had 'done wrong'. Further conversation revealed what was, in this particular moral context, an additional complicating factor: Nobisa did not love the father of the unborn child, and did not want to stay in a relationship with him. 'It was just a mistake', she said. At this point in the interview, her father became angry, asking what kind of girl would sleep with a boy she didn't even love.

Interestingly, it became evident that Nobisa's 13-year-old sister, Thandi, did not quite see things in the same way, although she strug-gled to articulate precisely what she thought. When I asked her what she thought about what was going on in her family, she looked at the floor and quietly replied: 'I just love my sister'. I understood this state-ment to mean that she supported her sister, and I wondered if she thought that, at that point in their lives, Nobisa was on the receiv-ing end of a lot of critical judgement, but not much love. It occurred to me that 13-year-old Thandi might not be a full member of that constitutive community which shaped up and imposed a moralizing and problem-saturated account of Nobisa's character. Thandi managed, through her simple and shyly made statement, to highlight Nobisa's aloneness, and thereby to make visible the moralizing judgements she was experiencing. I see this as a version of resistance, making visible what was otherwise not so easy to see. The stark difference between this brief statement of love, on the one hand, and the more pervasive attitudes of moralizing criticism, on the other, made the extent of the latter more visible. Nobisa's mother joined Thandi, and was next to undermine the hegemony of this moral discourse. Looking at Nobisa while Thandi struggled to speak, she said: 'I also love you my child'. It seemed to me that Thandi allowed her family to briefly assume a kind of distance from the judgemental, moralizing discourse that had captured them. Indeed, she had modelled such distance for them. Nobisa cried as this small gap appeared in the constitutive community of judgement, opening up a small crack through which the family could step, to begin to touch on different ways of orienting to this complex situation.

However, as already noted, a community's ways of being are not so easily overcome, and can make use of even the most loving and intimate of social partners to enforce its brief. A few minutes after the above interaction took place, Nobisa's father said: 'Yes, I love her too, of course', as he touched her gently on the shoulder. Then he turned to me and said:

> But let's not forget what Nobisa has done. I don't know if she has prayed for forgiveness, for the child who might have to grow up without a father, without a solid family, and for the hurt she has caused after all we've done for her. I don't think she realizes the full impact of this.

In the face of resistance – that is, a new potential discourse opening up through Thandi's (perhaps unintended) intervention – the constitutive community, the enforcers of the discourse, summons one of its most reasonable, authoritative, and well-placed agents: Nobisa's father, who lovingly reminds her, and everyone else, of her moral duty. 'Yes, everybody loves her', he seems to be saying, 'but that is not the issue; the *real* issue is her Christian morality'. 'I'm sorry daddy', Nobisa replied to her father's intervention. And so she is pulled back into her discursively appropriate, designated position, but in the most genuinely loving of ways.

There are four points I want to make with this case.

First, what I have termed the community of subjection is both a discursive achievement as well as a powerful enforcer of the values, ideals, and norms of the very discourses that constitute it: it is both product and vehicle. The local Christian community that plays such a powerful role in Nobisa's current circumstances is not a self-created community. They are the product of the long, complex, and sometimes geographically and culturally specific histories of Christianity into which they have been recruited. As such this specific community is a product of this discourse. But at the same time, their recruitment has them acting as its representatives. They monitor and police activities in the interests of sustaining its practices and values. It is within such a network of surveillance that Nobisa finds herself, and is encouraged to make sense of her life, her identity, and her choices.

This is not to suggest that members of a constituting community are Machiavellian in their intentions, that they spy on their neighbours, or seek to nakedly repress or control others. Nor do I suggest that members of such a community consciously aim for the production of obedient subjects. More often its members are intentionally drawn to help people to belong, to overcome their problems, to experience the good life, to grow morally, and in this case, to follow the word of God. But, from the perspective of discursive recruits, the answers to these questions – How should I conduct myself morally? How should I repair my relationship with God? – are to be found nowhere else but within the truth-telling discourse itself. We tend to act in good faith as discursive recruits, and as members of our communities of subjection; which is another way of saying that we tend to obey the requirements of those discourses that claim us.

Second, constitutive communities do allow persons to make positional shifts. A constituted subject is always, even within the confines of the constituting discourse, able to be known, or to know himself or herself, in altered ways. But there are conditions to these changes, conditions which ensure that the discourse and its values are sustained and/or enhanced, rather than undermined. So while such a community might fix a person to a position deemed appropriate to his or her circumstances, the person is not usually doomed to this position. We should consider, that is, the rules of discursive transformation: the discursively legitimized ways in which a person might move from one position to another; from a negative, judged, painful position, for instance, to a more normatively accepted and approved one. For instance, Petra, whose romantic dreams were shattered when her husband cheated on her, can reasonably be repositioned *within* the discourse of romance when she finds a new partner, moving from broken-hearted to romantically attached once again.

Similarly, in Nobisa's case, we might wonder what kind of movement is afforded a 'loose and immoral' girl in the kind of discourse of Christian morality that constitutes the community in which she currently resides. But there is a limit to such transformative possibilities. Consider the plight of prisoners, incarcerated psychiatric patients, and black persons during the tyranny of Apartheid in South Africa: all of these persons were constructed as having qualities or characteristics which make their integration into a particular community impossible (although of course, a variety of new communities could spring up around these persons). Once positioned in such an exclusionary way, there is little a person can do to reclaim his or her membership in the constituting community.

Might this apply in Nobisa's case? Might being a 'loose and immoral' girl be so deeply devalued a position that it warrants her exclusion from some aspect, or even all aspects, of this community's life? The fact that her family sought therapy suggested to me that this was not their intention. I had a sense that the family, at least, felt it possible for Nobisa to reclaim her position as a proper member of their Christian community. 'Forgiveness' seemed to play an important role within the Christian discourse represented by her family, and this might be one possible pathway to allow Nobisa to remain a full member of this configuration of community. But this is likely only to work on certain conditions; for instance, that she demonstrate an appreciation and appropriation of the correct values. Perhaps, then, in terms of the rules of this 'club', she could apologize profusely, acknowledge her guilt, experience the required shame, pray for forgiveness, and vow to learn from her mistakes. These are the kinds of requirements of the discourse, and its local enforcing community, for her to be recognized and valued as a fellow member.

Third, the constituting community itself is a powerful tool for the invisibilization of power. Some of the features of power's concealment, discussed in Chapter 2, can be clearly seen in operation in this case. We see how the labelling of Nobisa as a 'loose and immoral' individual draws attention away from the social forces that uphold such interpretations and hold Nobisa and her family to them. Our gaze is drawn to her personal failings, which seem to be the cause of her family's shame and the triggers of the community's seemingly reasonable negative judgements: 'What does she expect', a subject of this community might reasonably ask, 'she brought this on herself; she only has herself to blame!' We hear also that the moralizing Christian discourse has been naturalized as the only true way of making sense of the situation.

And in the interaction around Thandi's declaration of love for her sister, we notice the disqualification of other ways of orienting to Nobisa's situation. Thandi's intervention starkly highlighted the degrading and alienating effects of the moralizing environment: we should remember that while power tends towards invisibility, resistance can bring it to our notice. But Thandi's intervention is nevertheless easily constructed as naïve. Well meaning and sweet; it is even true – 'Yes, I love her too, of course'. But it is not, in many community members' eyes, up to the task of fully capturing the significance of the situation.

With this succession of tactics of invisibilization, an observer might declare that power has little to do with this situation: it's just a girl who made a terrible mistake and a caring family struggling to cope with its implications. Again, such a reading effectively conceals the host of power relations at play.

And my fourth point: the case illustrates that power is able to recuperate resistances and in the process 'learn' to improve its strategic operations. The role of resistance in power dynamics is by no means straightforward. Thandi's statement of love can be seen as a kind of resistance against the hegemonizing qualities of the powerful moralizing discourse circulating in the room. Not an intentional resistance – I do not assume she was deliberately trying to undermine the validity of her parents' or the broader community's views – but a resistance in the sense that it threatens to shift the accent of power just enough to diminish the force of the more moralistic position being adopted. In principle, effective resistances can disrupt power and usher in new discourses. However, Thandi's statement did not have this effect in the end, despite its promising beginnings. Her father listened to her, acknowledged his love for Nobisa, and then returned to the theme of shame – 'let's not forget what Nobisa has done...'. Instead of judging, shaming, and criticizing, Thandi's resistance leads her father to add a new, vital ingredient: now he judges, shames, and criticizes *with love*. Significantly, in the process, the discourse and practice of Christian morality are not simply *applied*, but are refined and advanced. Thandi's father does not just reinstate the original terms of the discussion, but alters it enough to make his criticism more palatable. The alienating effects of the situation, effectively exposed by Thandi's declaration of love, are softened.

One advantage of power's subtle responsivity – such as we see in Nobisa's father's slightly altered response – is that it can sometimes be enough to recuperate wayward subjects and justify its continued operation. In the case of Nobisa, the small shift in her father's talk might be enough to allow her to move back into the prevailing discourse and its values and practices. Indeed, her reply – 'I'm sorry daddy' – is in keeping with this. But we should recognize that in this instance, resistance *serves* power, rather than truly threatens it. It is less a case of a new discourse being introduced in response to Thandi's intervention, than it is of the old one being enhanced through it. One implication of this is that as communities encounter resistance to their ways of being, they sometimes evolve new strategies or techniques to advance the standing of their values and practices.

A subject whose alternative knowledges are disqualified

We saw in Chapter 2, and in Nobisa's case above, that one of the ways in which power is concealed is through the disqualification of alternative knowledges. When we discussed this point in Chapter 2, we were concerned with the occlusion of certain culturally available ways of thinking (e.g., discourses of gender equality) by other more prominent cultural discursive practices (e.g., of romance). In this section, I wish to consider the more personal ways in which this plays out, and to note how certain knowledges and experiences of life can be invisibilized by persons' positioning within powerful problem-saturated stories.

We have seen that knowledge and power coordinate to produce subjects into being. But in order to do so, it is necessary for alternative ways of knowing – and the alternative subject positions they make possible – to be disqualified or somehow minimized. It is clear that some ways of knowing become widely accepted and taken for granted in persons' lives. Some knowledges are designated as 'truth' or are culturally idealized, such as Petra's expectations around romantic love, and Oscar's understandings of masculinity. But we can trust that in the person's life there will always be 'subjugated knowledges', which are 'local, discontinuous, disqualified, illegitimate' (Foucault, 1980c, pp. 82–83).

One of Foucault's major contributions, taken on in narrative therapy, is his rejection of the idea that disqualified understandings are intrinsically inferior. Such a troubling of the authority of expert discourse is one of the primary ways in which Foucault follows Nietzsche, for whom the primary task of the philosopher was to 'create the conditions for indigenous spontaneity and to legitimate its products' (Smith, 1996, p. 163). We have seen – for example when discussing the disqualification of wise and experienced 'lay' persons through the valorization of expert psy discourses – that spontaneous indigenous knowledges are often designated as inferior by more dominant knowledge practices. Consider also Foucault's provocative question of the scientist: 'What types of knowledge do you want to disqualify in the very instant of your demand: "Is it a science?" Which ... subjects ... do you want to "diminish" when you say "I am a scientist"?' (1980c, p. 85). Likewise, the cultural valorization of 'real men', of 'coping under fire', of 'being strong', of 'being smarter than the next person', of 'the good girl', and so on, involve disqualifications or disparagements of different ways of being or knowing. Let us imagine Oscar, taking after Foucault's fiery resistance, putting the question to his father: 'What ways of knowing and being are you disqualifying when you say I am not "a real man"?' Any substantive answer to this question might take us to what is devalued, and through that to important unique outcomes in Oscar's life: as yet silenced or invisibilized ways of knowing and being that are not in line with the requirements of hegemonic masculinity. However, as a being constituted in and by a particular discourse of masculinity, Oscar cannot yet envisage such a question or the possibilities it offers.

The constituted subject then is, in part, that figure who has been recruited into performing his or her life in accordance with particular knowledge forms, and whose access to alternative knowledges and experiences – which have the potential to serve as a platform for unique outcomes and alternative story development – has become somehow limited, because they seem irrelevant, inapplicable, unrealistic ('pipe dreams'), untrue, naïve, or simply 'not me'. In my experience, clients sometimes speak of these other, disqualified experiences and ways of knowing as 'fluffy', as 'lacking depth', as promoting 'a denial of the real issues', or as 'wishful thinking'. We saw above, for example, that Nobisa's sister's comments and their potential effects – to create a more loving than critically moralizing atmosphere around Nobisa – were constructed as true but naïve; not up to the task of really capturing what was going on. Similarly, Oscar's hope that his father would support his questioning of all that had happened to him came to be seen as a naïve 'pipe dream'. It is all very well for me to invite Oscar to think about other ways of being a man or a human being, but these alternatives remain interpretable in problem-saturated ways in accordance with the dictates of masculine discourse.

Still, both Oscar and Nobisa's sister, Thandi, reveal other ways of knowing, doing, and being in the worlds they occupy. To members of their respective communities of subjection, including to some extent Oscar and Thandi themselves, these knowledges might seem limited or naïve. But such disqualified actions, hopes, expressions, and ways of knowing are significant for us as therapists because they are, to use White's phrase, 'out of phase' (2007, p. 61) with the requirements of the stories and practices that threaten to capture experience. They offer hope and create fractures in the forces of constitution to reveal something of profound importance: agency.

Moving towards agency

In this and the previous chapter, we have been exploring some of the contours of the Foucauldian constitutionalist perspective that informs narrative practice. This is a perspective that has been vigorously challenged for its apparent foreclosure of a coherent theoretical account of personal agency and resistance. But against such critiques, we have already seen some glimpses of the possibility of personal agency as emerging from within the constitutionalist account. In particular, we have seen that the notion of the person as not merely a product but also a vehicle of power attributes to the individual some minimal capacity to stand firm – albeit in subjected ways – as the winds of discourse blow around him or her. And we noted that power arrangements are formed among the multiplicity of constituting discourses, such that some enjoy wide circulation and support in particular communities and social practices, while others are disqualified or subjugated. For the narrative practitioner, these latter knowledges hold considerable promise, as they might enable resistance against imposed forces of constitution, and thereby point to a form of personal agency.

Let us turn now to examine in more depth the spaces the constitutionalist perspective opens up for resistance.

4

A Constitutionalist Account of Resistance

Clearly, for the narrative therapist the constituted subject can only be a partial description of the person. But such descriptions have considerable experiential thickness. Oscar's sense of himself as 'a failure', Petra's sense of herself as 'a stupid romantic', and Nobisa's personal sense of shame, for example, are all experienced as somehow central to their lives, evidencing an experiential depth and solidity that should be taken seriously. Nevertheless, it is evident that in practice narrative therapists embrace a more active vision of the human being than this constitutionalist picture makes available. The question of theory, however, is more complex, and it is by no means straightforward to assert that Foucault or White offer coherent theoretical grounds for such an active view.

In the next two chapters I will build the argument that the person is always able to refuse or otherwise unsettle the forces of constitution. I begin by discussing the position, represented by White and Foucault, that agency should be seen as a social rather than individual achievement: a product of the dynamics and complexities of person constitution, rather than something the individual is able to effect *as an individual*; in an extra-discursive, asocial manner. With the aid of some case material, I will then outline some of the limitations of this thoroughly social view, and in the following chapter propose a view of agency as grounded in what O'Leary (2002), in his studies on Foucauldian ethics, has described as the 'human animal' (p. 118). This is not intended to undermine the social ontological position as such, but rather to highlight that it can offer only a partial account of human agency. Indeed, it has been convincingly argued that Foucault's social formulations rely upon something like this human animal, without whom social power dynamics could not properly function (e.g., Falzon,

1993). And yet this figure is invisible not only in much of Foucault's work, but also in narrative therapeutic literature and theorizing. In this chapter and the next, I try to articulate the theoretical validity and therapeutic utility of this way of understanding the individual who is in some measure constituted, but not determined, by the social.

I would like to make some preliminary remarks about Foucault's position on agency and resistance, because this contributes a great deal to our understanding of certain key concepts in narrative practice. For example, the notions of 'unique outcomes' (White and Epston, 1990) and 'the absent but implicit' (Carey, Walther, and Russell, 2009), rely on the idea that the person is never a fully constituted subject, and nudge us towards the discovery and narration of those gaps in constitution that allow for alternative developments in the person's life.

Foucault was committed to a social ontological position (Hoy, 2004), meaning that he insisted on social rather than individual explanations of human conduct. As such, he stood in opposition to the naïve humanist belief in the autonomous, sovereign subject. But this does not mean he advocated social or discursive determinism. Foucault maintained that we have to move away from the idea that our ideas – and our selves – are 'no more than wind', blown around by discourse (in Veyne, p. 97). These winds are powerful, and they do blow us around to some extent, but in the end we can resist them. And it is here – in the belief in the individual's capacity to resist the winds and whims of discourse – that we find in Foucault the beginnings of an account of human agency. The reasoning is that if we can resist power, then at some level we can assume a capacity for agency. The ability to say 'no' is, for Foucault (1997b), only 'the minimal form of resistance' (p. 168). It can only be its starting point. And yet it implies a capacity for self-direction, and rescues us from being determined by the discourses and communities which shape us, and which blow us from here to there in our lives. So in order to understand human agency I begin with the question of resistance.

From the outset, I have tried to stress that there seems to be a contradiction in the very notion of resistance. How can Foucault maintain on the one hand a social ontological position, with its strong constitutionalist take on the subject, while on the other hand promoting what appears to be a somewhat more individualistic (and some (e.g., Wolin, 2006) say humanistic) perspective, in which he advocates persons' capacity to resist such constitution? Should he not, as Fish (1999) has suggested, have repudiated his earlier ideas of the subject as a product of discourse and power? These are good and fair questions to ask, and I wonder if they are asked enough in the narrative therapy universe.

Pinning down Foucault's stance on this theoretical tension is a complex, and perhaps ultimately impossible, task. I say this first because it is on the basis of this tension that some of the greatest philosophical and sociological minds of our time (e.g., Jurgen Habermas, Slavoj Žižek, Edward Said, Charles Taylor) see Foucault as presenting an incoherent and unworkable perspective on the questions of power, resistance, and agency. If it is hard for us to figure it out, we should console ourselves that we are in very good company. And if Foucault was 'horrified' at such apparent misreadings of his works, as Veyne (2010) tells us, we could be forgiven for wondering why he did not make it clearer.

Furthermore, it may be impossible to clarify what Foucault 'really' meant, or what his 'final' stance was, because we cannot make the assumption that his oeuvre should be read as a coherent whole. Foucault (1984) himself, in an essay entitled 'What is an author?', questioned the conventional practice of expecting ongoing coherence in written work simply because it is written by the same individual; as if the author was a coherent, self-contained, self-identical figure, somehow different from the rest of us. Can we assume that the Foucault of *The Archeology of Knowledge* or *The Birth of the Clinic* is at one with the Foucault who wrote *The History of Sexuality?* Is it reasonable to assume that they all add up to something like the 'final' Foucault? The problem, for us, is that while Foucault's earlier power/knowledge formulations are well developed and articulated, it is by no means clear how resistance – specifically, the resisting subject – fits in with that picture. This notion of resistance only emerged as a serious consideration later in his life. Some find solace in Foucault's (e.g., 1982) attempts, towards the end of his career, to argue that all of his different works are of a piece, each offering a different emphasis on the three pillars of our socio-historical existence that concerned him throughout: power, knowledge, and the subject (and its capacity for resistance). But for many critics, who saw the emergence of ideas like resistance, freedom, and creativity as unconvincing, superficial, and at odds with his earlier work on power/knowledge, this did not solve the problem.

Gutting (1994) is sceptical of Foucault's late attempt to graft coherence onto his life's work: is this a case of retrospective storying on Foucault's part; a kind of re-authoring in favour of a preferred, coherent self-narrative? Gutting essentially sides with Foucault's own critiques of the notion of the single-storied, self-contained author, and maintains instead that each of Foucault's works should be considered an independent piece of research. The upshot of Gutting's position is that it offers some support for Foucault's critics' view that he does not offer a definitive, coherent account of the relationship between power and resistance. The difference between Gutting and the critics, though, is that Gutting does not think he should have been expected to do so. But there is another side to this. There is agreement among many of Foucault's sympathizers (e.g., Deleuze, 1990; Falzon, 1993; Heller, 1996; Veyne, 2010) that there is more consistency to the Foucauldian project than such critiques and observations suggest. One just has to work a little harder, and perhaps read his works a little more sympathetically, to appreciate this. Specifically, on the question of the relationship between power and resistance, persons close to Foucault hold that he always at least implicitly marked out resistance as an important component – even a constitutive element – of power relations (Veyne, 2010). He might have made resistance explicit only a long time after publishing and lecturing on the different elements of power/knowledge, but the thought of it was always already there.

I want to acknowledge these debates about the coherence of Foucault's project(s) for one main reason: in narrative practice we tend to speak very freely about 'personal agency', despite the fact that our view of the social world tends to be shaped by Foucault's vision of power/knowledge dynamics (c.f., Besley, 2002). How can we do so? Habermas, Said, Žižek, and many others cannot see how these two dimensions of understanding come together. So is there something we know that they don't? As already mentioned, the answer is not to be found by clarifying what Foucault 'really' meant. This is not the issue for us. Perhaps his sympathizers, too, are not concerned so much with trying to read Foucault's mind, and do not assume that his works stand as the systematic unfolding over several decades of a single, preformed vision. We don't need to fight with Gutting. Perhaps we should instead be more concerned to build a coherent picture that need not be Foucault's, but which can be considered 'Foucauldian' in the sense that it builds on or is at least consistent with the foundational notion of power/knowledge. In any case, this is the stance I adopt here: I seek to contribute to building a theoretical formulation of the person as one who is constituted in and by power/knowledge dynamics, but who at the same time has a capacity for resistance and agency. My hope is that this might contribute to the tasks of narrative practice.

Where does resistance come from?
A constitutionalist account

What do we mean by resistance? This is a vitally important question for the post-structurally oriented narrative practitioner. As we shall see, it speaks to the heart of the issue of who is sitting across from us when we begin our narrative consultations. And yet it is a question whose answer I feel is still to be clarified. The nub of the issue is this: if there is no sovereign, authorial, centred subject, then *who* is doing the resisting? What is the basis of the person's resistance, if not the very autonomous, choosing, sovereign subject that both Foucault and White have already rejected? This problem haunted Foucault and continues to divide commentators on his work to this day. As Deleuze (1990), speaking of Foucault, put it: 'It was all very well to invoke points of resistance as "counterparts" of foci of power, but where was such resistance to come from?' (p. 98).

Foucault's original constitutionalist position would not permit a view of resistance as emerging from the individual himself or herself; as emerging from pre-existing (e.g., biological or characterological) abilities, skills, inclinations, predispositions, or wisdoms. If, as narrative practitioners, we take the position that there is no a priori self (c.f., Madigan, 2010), then such a figure cannot stand as author or originator of this resistance. The belief in a pre-existing self, which lies behind or beneath the narrative, threatens to collapse our thinking into essentialism and naturalism. So, in answer to the question – Is there some essential, inherent, natural, human force, instinct, or principle that instigates resistance; that 'tells' us what to resist and what to accept; that guides us 'from within' on what social prescriptions and norms to obey and which to refuse? – Foucault gives us an emphatic 'no'. This would seem to leave us in the strange position of accepting that our resistance to the forces of power, or social constitution, emerges from those very social forces themselves. Do we believe that our forms of constitution initiate and drive our resistance against our forms of constitution? Must we accept such a constitutionalist account of resistance? Well, there is indeed some validity to this view, insofar as our constitution in multiple discourses means we can draw from one to challenge another (as we shall discuss in more detail below). But I will argue that this answer is not satisfactory as an overall understanding, and we need not limit ourselves to it, despite White and Foucault's apparent allegiance to that view.

So let us examine what I perceive to be three of the main strands of the constitutionalist view of resistance.

The failure of power

The first can be identified via Michael White's (2004) utilization of Foucault's idea that power is never fully successful:

If systems of power are very rarely total in their effects, and if the operations of ... power are everywhere to be perceived, then examples of opposition to the relations of modern power, or of actions that represent a refusal of its requirements, will be ever present.

(White, 2004, p. 155)

On this account, resistance is possible because discourse, or the power/knowledge dynamic, never succeeds completely in making human beings into its subjects. Power is incomplete. Thus, for instance, the diagnoses of schizophrenia and dependent personality disorder, the labels 'loser', 'failure', 'incompetent', and 'worthless', are never sophisticated enough, comprehensive enough, operationalized effectively enough, or taken up by enough social participants in sufficiently aligned ways, to completely capture the people they try to describe. Oscar's sense of himself as a failure, for example, cannot encapsulate the whole of his being or experience. White's argument here is not that if the person opposes power it will not always work. Rather, his position is the reverse: if power does not always work, then the person will resist it. The person here is not seen to embody some excess that can never be contained by social discourse and power dynamics. Rather, to put it crudely, the person can resist not because he or she is strong and capable, but because power is weak and fragmented.

Illustrating this view, White (2004) tackles the sense of 'personal failure', which he feels everyone experiences at some point in their lives. This phenomenon, he notes, emerges when the person is recruited to perform his or her life 'according to the constructed norms of culture' (p. 154), but then is unable to measure up to them. Not everyone can realize the ideals to be found in a particular culture: not everyone can be the winner or the leader, a genius, manly, beautiful, moral, thin, or independent. White then argues, in an interesting twist, that this failure to measure up is not a personal failure, but 'an example of the *failure* of modern power itself' (p. 174; emphasis added). Simply put, White's view is that power fails when it does not manage to turn us into the ideals it prescribes for us. On this basis, a range of apparently personal failures – such as Oscar's sense of being a weak man – can be re-characterized as 'feats of opposition to modern power, or as acts of refusal of what is being required by it' (White, 2004, p. 175).

White's stance is reminiscent of the feminist stance Orbach (1978) took (albeit from a different perspective) regarding the positioning of women in relation to gender stereotypes in certain societies. Against the idealizations of the thin woman, Orbach argues that 'getting fat' should be seen as 'a definite and purposeful act' (p. 31) of rebellion against prevailing images of the ideal woman and standards of beauty. Similarly, Chernin (1981) sees anorexia and obesity in terms of women's 'unexpressed hostility' and 'uneasiness about what is expected of women in this culture' (p. 73). While White would not put things in terms such as 'unexpressed hostility', there seems to be a synergy between these perspectives, consisting in the view that (1) power is unable to turn everyone into its ideal subjects, and (2) this failure positions certain subjects as resistant. This is not to say that the person's resistance is triggered, 'allowed', or given space, by power's failure. It is not that power's failure makes visible a fracture in its systems, allowing us to act on our already existing desire to escape. The view here seems to be that power's failure itself *produces* non-conforming subjects. We are resisters not necessarily because we want to resist, or have chosen to resist, but because power fails to sculpt us to its specifications, making us somehow Other. We thereby, albeit unwittingly, stand as examples of alternative ways of being.

I will argue below that there are problems with this account (and also that the sense of personal failure that White (2004) refers to is a problematic example both of resistance and of the failure of modern power). But for now, let us move on to the second aspect of the constitutionalist account of resistance.

Social models of resistance

The second aspect of the constitutionalist perspective is that we learn to resist via exposure to what Foucault (1997d) refers to as 'models' for resistance found in the 'culture' (p. 291). This is the answer White (2004) seems to arrive at after posing the very question with which we are concerned: 'What is the foundation of... refusal?', he asks: 'What is it that makes... refusal possible?' (p. 175). The meaning of his explicit answer to this question is less than clear (at least to me), but I wish to mention it nonetheless. After asserting that resistance cannot come from some essential, authentic, natural, core self, he goes on to say that his answer to this question is

> informed by the observation that if a person is refusing to live the life that s/he is assigned to live, and is not being the person whom s/he is required to be, then s/he is living a different life and is being someone else, whom s/he might not have significantly been before – that s/he is pursuing some alternative identity projects that

do not so comprehensively reproduce the norms for the favoured individualities of our culture.

(White, 2004, pp. 176–177)

What is one to make of this answer? White is telling us that resistance is there when the person does not totally perform certain cultural norms, and is instead living in ways that deviate from these norms. In this answer he seems to effectively credit the person with an already existing *alternative* life, narrative, and identity project. But this begs the question: where did these alternatives come from?

For White, the person's alternative storylines are ultimately social products. The 'foundation for…opposition' (White, 2004, p. 186) lies, it seems, in the person's expressions of what matters most to him or her in terms of values, principles, or ethics; these too must be discursive products. They refer to the person's location or positioning in some 'different' (i.e., nonproblem-saturated) discourse that has taken hold somewhere else in the person's life. He offers a case example of a woman named Judy, who has been in the grip of the demands of the self-help culture, which tell her that she must become independent and competent in order to have a fulfilling life. Having failed to achieve these goals, Judy experiences herself as dependent and incompetent. But White also notices that she does not fully subscribe to these descriptions. In the therapeutic dialogue, it emerges that she places a high value on an 'ethic of partnership' (2004, p. 186), which celebrates her tendency to collaborate with others, and thereby makes available a counter discourse to those constructions of her actions in terms of a failure of independence.

We have to read this account carefully to find out where White sees the origins of her resistance (i.e., resistance against descriptions of herself as dependent and incompetent), because he does not tell us. To avoid an essentialist and naturalist position, White indicates that he cannot argue that Judy's opposition to stories of her dependency and incompetence is based somehow on the idea that this is not who she 'really is', or that dependency and incompetence are socially learned impositions that distort her innate drive to self-fulfilment or personal growth. And, of course, he certainly cannot claim that an ethic of partnership is a built-in, a priori desire of the human being as such. But he does suggest that a story of such partnership is already there, not inbuilt, but woven into her life via exposure to such partnering performances by others. Reading through the case we discover that Judy may have learned aspects of this way of being from her Aunt Clara, who also demonstrated a relational ethic.

We will return to this case below, but for now we note that power's failure produces non-conforming subjects, and the person's ability to purposefully adopt the consequent non-conformist, resisting stance, depends on social learnings and exposure to other ways of being. On this point, White joins with Foucault, who put it this way:

> these (active, resisting) practices are...not something invented by the individual himself. They are models that he finds in his culture and are proposed, suggested, imposed upon him by his culture, his society, and his social group.
>
> (Foucault, 1997d, p. 291)

Reinforcing this stance, White noted that narrative practices are often misunderstood on the question of agency: the person's preferences, intentions, identity claims, and indeed resistances, are all based on historical and cultural forms, rather than on any internal 'essence', or 'element' 'to be "found" at the centre of who one is' (White, 2004, p. 129). We have no choice but to make meaning out of the 'materials lying about in society' (White, 2004, p. 103); materials which in Judy's case include impressions and experiences of her Aunt Clara. This view concludes then that one's impulse to resist, and one's rationale for such action (e.g., founded on a learned 'ethic of partnership'), do not stem from the inside, but ultimately from the outside.

The lure of discourse

The third way in which resistance emerges can be identified via what Veyne (2010) calls the 'lure' of discourse (p. 114).

We can be assured of the existence of alternative discourses. This is because we exist in a multiply constructed world, in which there are a virtually endless number of alternative discursively constructed ways of being. In White's (2000) words, 'people live out their lives in various contexts or zones...in which different identity claims are verified' (p. 7). These different 'contexts or zones' carry different discourses, which according to discourse theorists Laclau and Mouffe (2001), operate in a strategic field of social antagonisms. As already discussed, each discourse strives towards the centre of particular social spaces, to have its own truths represented in social practice, and so must contend with others competing for the same interpersonal zones or contexts. For this to work, each discourse must have its lures, its tactics of enticement and promise; each must have some sort of reasonable, plausible, attractive grounds for our positioning within them.

On this account, which relies both on power's inability to be totalizing in its effects, and on the existence of social and cultural models for resistance, resistance can result from the subjectifying or home-providing powers of an *alternative* discourse, and the communities it offers. For example, power's inability to turn Judy into its ideal – the 'independent and competent' person – made space for an alternative formulation. And this alternative – the ethic of partnership – no doubt appealed to Judy: White showed his own support for this discourse, understanding it to be something aligned with Judy's preferences, and together they found a kind of embodied nodal point for it in Judy's Aunt Clara. It also at least implicitly promised a different and less problem-saturated way of being. Of course, the problem constituting discourse also has its own lures: its ways of fighting back. The self-help promises of personal fulfilment and competence can be very attractive indeed. To take another example, it is not hard to see that Oscar (who felt a failure as a man) might resist attempts to redefine his existence in terms dissociated from masculinity, because hegemonic masculinity is able to offer powerful lures for him to remain in its grasp (e.g., to be admired as a masculine man). But when he does resist these lures and speaks out against his abuse, it might be the case that he has become subject to the enticements of an alternative discourse: the promise that he can finally 'be himself', perhaps, or the suggestion that if he 'lets it out', rather than holding on to his shameful secret, he might experience a sense of liberation. But then we saw, via his father's judgemental response, how he was lured back into hegemonic masculinity – this time, not by a promise of something better, but via a reminder of his masculine duty to face his failures 'as a man'.

In any event, with respect to the issue of resistance, the proposal here is that a new discourse and its models can lure the person away from the prevailing discursive or narrative universe, and thereby potentially activate resistances against it. This new discourse is not objectively 'better' – we can make no such judgement as post-structural thinkers – but perhaps at certain key moments its subjectifying or hailing qualities – its lures – become more effective. This new set of subject positions equips persons to resist the prevailing discursive arrangements. All discourses have lures, but it is when gaps or failings appear in the prevailing discourse that lures to alternate spaces of living become more persuasive, and their subjectifying potentials are increased.

The three factors associated with this constitutionalist position on resistance – power's failure, social models, discursive lures – are obviously interrelated. In the first instance, the incompleteness of power makes room for alternative discourses to fill up these gaps, errors, or slippages; these alternative discourses contain their own promises, offerings, and solicitations, and lure the person away from their original positions; and certain social and cultural models provide different scripts as well as enabling communities and social practices to further support resisting actions. This is a thoroughgoing social constitutionalist perspective, which rests on a view of agency as a socially constituted rather than an individual product.

Let us consider, with a more detailed case example, how such a perspective might inform our understandings of the persons who consult us.

A case illustration: Devri's escape from abuse

I met with Devri, a 27-year-old woman who was in what sounded like an abusive relationship with her husband, Raj. Devri was referred by her medical practitioner for 'depression and anxiety', and in his referral letter he noted that there were 'marriage problems'. Devri came in alone, since Raj refused to take part in therapy. She told me that Raj had beaten her on several occasions, and she felt controlled by him. She said that Raj 'acts like he owns me, like I'm his *thing*'. She said that she had had enough and wanted to leave him, but at the same time she was experiencing considerable ambivalence around this. She longed for the freedom a divorce would bring, but feared this would bring shame on herself and her family. She explained that in her culture and religion, a woman leaving her husband creates a shameful reputation not only for her, but also for her whole family.

How should we conceptualize Devri's desire to leave the relationship and end the abuse she was suffering? How to conceptualize her resistance? In terms of the constitutionalist position, as we have seen, this desire to leave the abusive relationship cannot be seen as 'natural'. It cannot be seen as a product of some innate, pre-given, animal-like instinct, drive, or need: such as to avoid pain, to have space to express one's individuality, to be 'free', or even to protect oneself from assault. Foucault (1997a) argued that even the will to not be controlled should not be considered 'an originary aspiration' (p. 75). Even this is something we must learn about (or not) through social modelling and exposure to cultural and other narratives.

Thus, Devri's resistance to being physically and emotionally abused must, according to this constitutionalist account, be associated in some way with the three processes mentioned above. First – in line with White's (2004) belief that 'systems of power are very rarely total in their effects' (p. 155) – there must be some failure of the locally controlling narrative and associated practices, which (i.e., this failure) positions Devri as non-conformist. Mindful of White's (2004) arguments around the issue of personal failure, we might imagine that her 'failure' to live up to the standards required of a wife in her cultural and religious context not only reflects the relative failure of these discourses to fully recruit her into the values, ideals, and models they prescribe for her life, but also immediately positions her as non-compliant; as resistant. Power can also fail in a relational sense. Devri's husband, Raj, could not oversee all of her activities, and the regulatory community of which she is part is not as uniform in its gendered approach to marriage as might be supposed. These enforcers of power could not, for instance, always monitor her conversations with other women, with whom she had discussed her difficult situation. Raj's control of her, despite its far-reaching effects in her life, is necessarily incomplete. Likewise, the cultural and familial prescriptions for women's relationships with men do not extend to every corner of her life, to her every thought or feeling. Even the shame prescribed for herself and her family – should she leave him – would not consume every aspect of their lives. On this account, power simply does not have the full resources of perfect social alignment, observation, monitoring, and enforcement to ensure Devri's, or her family's, total compliance with its requirements.

Second, Devri must have available to her alternative cultural and social models which problematize abuse and/or support different ways of being. For instance, in response to some questions, she told me that in conversation with friends she heard about other women who had removed themselves from abusive situations, invoking notions of 'human rights' to build supportive narratives. Of course, she had always known about human rights, but it was not until our conversation that she began to think of her relationship in these terms. It frightened her to think about it this way, but it now became possible for her to imagine herself as one endowed with such rights. White's position here might be that she is now, at least in part, 'living a different life and is being someone else, whom she might not have significantly been before – that she is pursuing some alternative identity projects' (White, 2004, pp. 176–177). That is, we might assume that in some respects, as she engages with these social models – the women with whom she speaks, and the stories she hears – she tentatively begins to think of herself as not just an owned woman but as a human being with rights. In the process, as White might have it, Devri is already, albeit minimally, 'being someone else'; someone other than the controlled 'thing' she had become.

And third, we might envision Devri being at the centre of a discursive tussle, wherein competing lures strive to entice her over to one or other way of living her life. The discourse of human rights, represented by the stories she hears from friends, and the characters within them, inscribes her with rights she did not fully realize that she had. It highlights not only that she can refuse to go on being abused, but also that she is entitled to think of herself not as an owned 'thing' but as a person endowed with the fundamental right to self-governance. These alternative ideas slip through the cracks of the never-fully sutured discourse of gendered power relations. And as they slip through, their lures – their promises of 'freedom' or 'liberation' – can begin to take on significance in Devri's thoughts. But we hear also of her ambivalence. The cultural discourses of devotion, loyalty in marriage, family honour, and so on, lure her in other ways. Remaining a devoted wife, for example, might give her legitimate standing in her sociocultural sphere. It gives her a powerful sense of belonging, in a way that discourses of human rights might not explicitly provide. Perhaps from this perspective, the adoption of human rights looks like a lonely and risky path to take. She is threatened with dishonour should she leave. Which lures will be most effective?

Thus, in accordance with the social constitutionalist perspective articulated above, we might theorize that her resistance is explained by (1) the failure of power (2) the availability of alternative role models and ways of thinking, and (3) the luring power of these alternatives. Devri's resistance is in other words constructed as a thoroughly social product.

However, this formulation has its problems, the articulation of which might prove useful in nuancing our understanding of resistance.

A critique of the constitutionalist position

Before critiquing this stance, we should note that neither Foucault nor White was an extreme constitutionalist at the end of the day. It is probably true that their theoretical discussions repeatedly and strongly support a constitutionalist perspective, with White drawing significantly on Foucault on this issue. But when one reads between the lines in both of their works – for example, when one reads Foucault's interviews and later lectures, or White's comments on agency, intentionality, and his conduct in therapeutic conversations – it becomes clear that both display a certain level of discomfort with the constraints of such a position. There is indeed something important in the constitutionalist account, and it affords some significant theoretical advantages – it prevents the slide into individualism, essentialism, naturalism, or naïve humanism. But it doesn't *quite* fit. It is as if both White and Foucault believed that the idea of the socially constituted subject reasonably outlines the effects of power/knowledge on the person's life, but also that it does not tell us the full story. This is the position I adopt here: we are constituted beings, but we are also more than this. The excess bit – the piece that doesn't quite fit with a wholly constitutionalist perspective – concerns precisely the issues of resistance and agency (and which I will take up in the next chapter). But I think that neither Foucault nor White really fleshed out that fuller story, theoretically speaking. And so it still remains unclear how either Foucault (e.g., Habermas, 1990) or White (e.g., Burnette, 1995) make sense of this apparent contradiction between the constituted subject – for which they have argued so thoroughly and persuasively – and the resisting/agentive subject – to which only more limited theoretical attention has been given. Nevertheless, this is the point at which we find ourselves: constitutionalists with an incomplete account of resistance and agency.

There exist multiple critiques of the constitutionalist position on power associated principally with Foucault's writings. I want to focus here on those that touch specifically on the issues of resistance and personal agency. There are four main challenges to note. The first is the observation that power's failure does *not* necessarily lead to resistance. Second, as Habermas (e.g., 1990) asks of Foucault, if power is intrinsically neither good nor bad (as we saw in Chapter 2), and if there are no foundational norms to stand behind, then why is resistance a good thing? Why should people bother? Third, the idea that resistance is a function of the luring capacities of discourse is limited in that it continues to construct human beings as passive, docile figures. And fourth, I problematize the Foucauldian requirement that social models are necessary for resistance. I will discuss these four points, before concluding that the strong constitutionalist position, consisting in the claim that personal agency or resistance is totally a social product, can only take us part of the way.

Power's failure does not necessarily lead to resistance

I want to begin by arguing, contra White (2004), that we should not automatically consider the sense of personal failure an example of power's failure, or as pointing to the fracturing of a particular discourse, in the first place. It seems to me that White conflates the *ideals* of a discourse (e.g., *being* thin, competent, a real man, a good wife) with the *values* associated with it (e.g., *striving* to be thin, competent, manly, a good wife). There is good reason to suggest that the failure to attain an ideal can be seen as evidence not of power's failure, as White would have it, but precisely of its success.

In this regard, we should note Foucault's (1977) argument that power works by situating persons within a normative *distribution* in a particular field of power relations. In this way, 'the power of normalization imposes homogeneity', although not in the sense that it makes everyone exactly the same (Foucault, 1977, p. 184). What is to remain the same – the homogeneity – is not the individuals within a normative field, or their achievements, but the rules, values, and ethos of the discourse. It is in the context of this homogeneity that normative power '*individualizes* by making it possible to measure gaps, to determine levels, to fix specialities and to render the differences useful by fitting them one to another' (Foucault, 1977, p. 184, emphasis added). For example, Foucault tells us that the discourses of normality describe 'a whole range of degrees of normality indicating membership of a homogeneous social body but also playing a part in classification, hierarchization and the distribution of rank' (p. 184). Thus, the power of the norm works not to make everyone attain the same high standards of good, competent, manly, thin, and so on, but to order, distribute, and rank people in terms of their achievements on such dimensions. It follows that the failure to achieve the loftiest standards – the sense of personal failure White describes – is not at all evidence of power's failure; it is already part of the plan.

Indeed, this kind of distribution (e.g., from dependent to independent; from strong man to weak man) is very often necessary for power's success. In Chapter 2, we encountered Sampson's (1993) argument that the adoption of culturally preferred positions (e.g., as 'rational') rests on 'serviceable others' being positioned in culturally undesirable ways (e.g., 'emotional'). The implication is that, within the context of a particular set of discursive practices, the person deemed a 'failure' stands as a kind of serviceable other, a contrasting background against which those deemed successful can be foregrounded. Foucault did not put it in Sampson's terms, but I see a congruence with the idea that discourses deploy norms to order, categorize, and to have people compare themselves with each other; all, ultimately, in the service of a particular power arrangement. Bluntly put, Judy's sense of being a personal failure (as incompetent and dependent) is at some level necessary for others to be positioned as successes (as competent and independent). Likewise, Oscar's sense of being not a real man is a necessary part of the overall discursive strategy of recruiting men to participate in reproducing the norms of masculinity. They should compete with each other to move up the ladder towards the normative ideal this discourse describes. Both real men, and those who fail to be real men, are necessary for the operations of hegemonic masculinity. Likewise, with respect to Orbachs' (1978) stance on 'fat' women, and Chernin's (1981) position on anorexia and obesity, it becomes problematic to hold up such experiences themselves as resistance (although, of course, they can *become* resistances through reframing, storying, or re-authoring interventions).

A final point on this issue: if we look at Michael White's work with Judy more closely, I think it is reasonable to suggest that he mislocates her resistance. This is an important issue, worthy of brief mention, because it highlights our need for an improved understanding of the origins of resistance. It seems to me that Judy's resistance did not lie so much in her 'failure' to attain certain normatively prescribed ideals – what White sees as her non-conformism – but in her assumption of a far more active position. At first, she describes trying all manner of strategies to reach these ideals, including the use of self-help books. In this respect, we could say that she was still recruited into maintaining the ideals of competence and independence, even if she was not yet high up in their ranks. She was still, in a manner of speaking, a compliant subject, obeying but failing to achieve the goals set for her. But, in the therapeutic conversation, the turning point comes when she says 'I've pretty well given up now' (White, 2004, p. 180). White is right, I think, to act on this as her moment of resistance, and in a pragmatic flash of genius he seizes on this moment and asks how she 'managed to step back' from those requirements (p. 180), and poses other questions to thicken this unique outcome. White sees a therapeutic opportunity in the fact that she hints at having given up on the normatively prescribed task into which she had formerly been recruited. But at a theoretical level he does not comment on the fact that her resistance lay not in her failure to live up to these ideals (which is what his discussion suggests), but in her desire to give up on the normative system which had sustained them in her life ('I've pretty well given up now'). In other words, she resists not by failing to meet certain standards, but by giving up on them. And because White theoretically insists on the former (i.e., failure as resistance), it remains unclear how Judy came to this resistance in the first place (we will turn to the social models supporting her resistance below).

It seems to me that the equation 'power's failure = resistance' misrecognizes the situation in Judy's case. Similarly, it would be misleading to suggest that Devri's resistance was a by-product of her not being totally subject to the discourses of gender relations prescribed in her cultural and religious milieu. Her resistance is not associated with her 'failure' to be a devoted wife (for instance), but with her objection to being controlled and treated as somebody's 'thing'. This is a more active resistance than White seems to suggest. My understanding of this is that the failure to live up to certain standards is not resistance per se, although with some work it can evolve into a kind of resistance, or intentional non-conformism.

My second critique of the 'power's failure = resistance' position White seems to put forward concerns the question: why would power's failure lead to resistance, and not some other outcome? Consider that discourses provide us with narrative and social 'homes'. Our constitution as subjects in a particular discursive arrangement is our very way of belonging, of being linked in with the world around us; it is our way of being knowable, and of coming to know ourselves. In terms of the constitutionalist perspective, then, surely we would be just as likely to support the fractured power system as to undermine it. As Judith Butler (1997) put it: 'To exist, we must submit to power. Then we come to desire our own submission, because it's better than not existing at all. Subjection is how the individual derives social intelligibility' (p. 6). In other words, we cannot assume, as White does, that power's imperfections lead to the omnipresence of 'examples of opposition to the relations of modern power, or of actions that represent a refusal of its requirements' (p. 155). Is White assuming that power is something we always wish to refuse? For the Foucauldian thinker, and White knew this well, the successful refusal of one form of power can, at best, lead only to its replacement with another or others. It would therefore be a mistake to think that a subjectified, successfully recruited soldier, psychiatric patient, abused woman, or type-A businessperson, would automatically rush to escape from their situations simply because the opportunity presented itself.

In the case of Judy we can assume that she would have had several opportunities to escape the problem-saturated stories of herself as incompetent and dependent. Perhaps she tried to take some of these opportunities; we cannot know. But in any case she comes into therapy, and is energized when talk focuses on her valuing of an ethic of partnership. She shows, at least here, some kind of intention to resist the old prescriptions and positions. But why does she *want* to do so? As one who has internalized or taken on the particular dictates of self-help and self-improvement discourses, is she not equally likely to fill these gaps, these failures of power, herself, further thickening and nuancing these discourses? After all, do they not already offer her a promising pathway forward? She might well heed the advice of Napoleon Hill, an early author in the personal-improvement and success genre: 'When defeat comes, accept it as a signal that your plans are not sound, rebuild those plans, and set sail once more toward your coveted goal' (2013, p. 92). Perhaps Judy could re-evaluate her efforts, try a new tactic, be more patient with herself, buy the latest self-improvement book, find a new guru, support group, or life coach, and steer herself once more in the desired direction. In other words, the fact that self-improvement discourse sometimes evidences holes, cracks, imperfections, and an inability to perfectly fulfil the promises it makes, does not explain why Judy would reject it. Surely under such circumstances, power's inefficiency could be forgiven, and lead not to resistance, but to reinvigorated subjection.

My point is that a gap in power will not *necessarily* lead to resistance, or even to a desire for resistance. A few years after I first qualified as a clinical psychologist, a friend and I were trying to introduce constructionist thought into our practices and peer-supervision meetings, and we had come across White and Epston's *Narrative Means to Therapeutic Ends*. At this time, I was referred a 30-year-old woman, Hannelie, who had recently been diagnosed with bipolar disorder. Inspired by the externalizing thinking expressed in White and Epston's classic text, I engaged in a conversation with her around the effects of this label on her hopes for her life. Now, I do not claim to have led this conversation very efficiently, and I made the rookie mistake of assuming that 'bipolar disorder' was an enemy to be defeated. Whatever my mistakes, it became evident to Hannelie that I was taking a critical position relative to psychiatric ways of thinking about her situation. So, on the one hand she was captured within the powerful psychiatric discourse in the form of a label that seemed to pathologize her. But on the other hand, she was faced with a qualified psychologist talking to her in a very different way, who refused to see her as psychiatrically disturbed, or mentally ill. My words, together with my status as a professional, the degrees on my wall, and so on, surely represented a legitimate fracturing of psychiatric power. I was 'officially' making open to her another way of thinking about her situation. If resistance issues from the gaps in power, then

I was trying to point to and hold open just one of these gaps. But she did not take it. Instead, she ended up getting rather annoyed and resorted to explaining to me the medical and biological 'facts' associated with her 'condition'. Sadly, she did not come for a follow-up meeting.

I like to think that I would handle this situation differently if it came up again, now that I have more experience. But this scenario nonetheless illustrates an important point. People often value their forms of subjection, even when they seem toxic in others' eyes. People do not resist power simply because they can, or because they are given permission to do so.

It is one thing to say that the prison, the hospital, the abusive marriage, stories of dependency, and other psychiatric diagnosing practices, 'fail' in the sense that each of them contains barely visible escape routes (physical or metaphorical). It is quite another to assume that the person will take them. We can agree with White (and Foucault) that power is not total in its effects. That might make room for resistance, but it does not explain its emergence. We still need to explain how it is, in the context of a specific power's inability to be everywhere at all times, that the person resists.

Why bother to resist?

Second, we have the question: why would we bother to resist if no story, no morality, no truth, no form of social order, is inherently superior to any other? This is the primary critique Habermas (1990) levels at the Foucauldian constitutionalist perspective. For Habermas, Foucault's refusal to say what is right and what is wrong, what should be supported and what resisted, makes his position hopelessly relativistic. We are left with no grounds on which to determine what counts as legitimate resistance. So, the Habermasian question goes, if we accept no 'normative foundations' (Habermas, 1990, p. 276), then why should people bother to resist at all? After all, the new place to which the resisting person moves is, theoretically speaking, neither better nor worse than the place he or she moved away from.

This is an important challenge for us: how do we know which resistances – Devri's against being owned, Judy's against self-improvement projects, or Oscar's against masculinity – to support, and which are erroneous or flawed? Habermas' implication is that our decisions in this regard matter from a political perspective: what kind of politics do our decisions and actions support? And why? In psychoanalysis, according to Habermas (1987), valid resistances – and hence, valid personal-political projects – can be distinguished from invalid ones.

The practitioner might interpret some client protests in terms of what Freud (1963) called 'legitimate dissent' (p. 262), while others might be seen as lacking in rational substance: as repetition compulsions, unconscious fantasies, defence mechanisms, and so on. Such distinctions are seen to aid the psychoanalyst in assisting persons' movement towards legitimate dissent, thereby enabling their engagement in unclouded, clear, rational, consensual communicative interaction. Such a move, according to Habermas, in turn allows persons to participate legitimately in societal power dynamics. In the end, for Habermas (1987), psychoanalysis thereby facilitates democratic process.

His accusation is that Foucault – and we should add the narrative therapist – has no means for distinguishing legitimate from illegitimate resistance, and hence no rationale for supporting one project over another. Indeed, our commitment to the social ontological and constitutionalist perspective means that our resistances lack normative grounds. In therapeutic practice, then, we cannot argue that a person resists because the situation he or she is in is 'morally wrong', based on 'lies' or 'misunderstandings', or deforming of his or her 'true self'. We cannot argue that the person resists because he or she does not want to face up to some hidden truth (as the psychoanalyst might); after all, we do not believe in any such underlying truths. And the post-structural narrative practitioner cannot hold that resistance draws persons from 'bad' forms of power to the 'good'. We simply have no absolute truths or moral standards to distinguish one from the other. Of course, in our therapeutic work we do sometimes promote or support certain kinds of resistances on the basis of social and historically specific values, understandings, and conditions. But this, I think, is part of Habermas' question: do we resist simply when the historical and social winds of discourse tell us to do so?

Habermas' astute critique comes to this: in Judy's case, our social ontology makes it difficult for us to assume any intrinsic superiority of the ethic of partnership over the culturally valorized story of striving for personal improvement. Both provide her with a potential 'place' from which to make sense of her situation, and we cannot assume that either would construct an a priori 'better' social system or way of being in the world. Likewise, in Devri's situation of abusive conflict in the home, on what basis can we argue that the human rights discourse is inherently better than the cultural and gendered discourses of heterosexual relationships that predominate in her life? And we have already seen in the case of Hannelie's diagnosis of bipolar disorder, that my preferences for a non-pathological view of her situation were rejected;

I naively thought one view was better, she evidently disagreed. Such preferences, at least on the constitutionalist account, have no absolute, transcendent standing. So on what grounds are our resisting preferences justified?

It is clear that Foucault did indeed take sides. He did not spend his time sitting on the fence, assuming the relativist position that all things are equal. Instead, in both his academic and personal life, he resisted a number of practices of power. Habermas (1990) recognized this apparent contradiction, and accused Foucault of adopting a 'cryptonormative' stance (p. 284): a position that rested on unacknowledged, disavowed norms. Foucault seemed to take the side of the so-called homosexual over the discourses privileging heterosexuality; of prisoners over the prison guards; of free speech over governed speech. Likewise, it is clear that White does not advocate neutrality in therapeutic work. With David Epston, he noted the implication of the Foucauldian position that we could not take a 'benign view of our practices' and that our involvement in power/knowledge dynamics, as participants rather than observers, was inevitable (White and Epston, 1990, p. 29). He was clearly opposed to some of the effects of modern power (e.g., White, 2004). Another obvious example of this can be seen in how David Epston and others take a clear side against anorexia and bulimia, and against the 'pro-ana' movement that supports these ways of being (e.g., Lock, Epston, Maisel, and de Faria, 2005). We take positions on certain things, and the therapeutic conversation is always 'politicized' in this sense. This is a direct implication of our belief in our immanence in a field of power relations: we cannot avoid power, and so if we are not to be pushed around by it, we must take a stand. But, in terms of Habermas' question, on what grounds we make these decisions is not quite so clear. Do we carry some invisible set of norms – a cryptonormativity – to justify our own, and our clients', resisting practices?

This is a complex field of debate to which I cannot do justice here (see, for example, King, 2009, for a fuller discussion on the Habermas–Foucault debate on normativity). But Habermas' critique merits attention. In response, I wish to begin by briefly outlining my position – to be developed further in Chapter 7 – that a certain approach to ethics can be used to inform our commitments. As Habermas (1993) himself asserts, one's personal or community ethics are fundamentally tied to 'the underlying question: "Who am I, and who would I like to be?" ("Who are we, and who would we like to be?")' (p. 127). The linkage of ethics with these questions is remarkably aligned with the position

Foucault takes in his later works, and with the position I advocate for narrative practice in later chapters. As I see it, however, our adoption of a post-structural Foucauldian position means that we cannot answer such questions for another person or community. We do not prescribe normative contents. We do not specify that this or that is the right way to live, nor do we indicate which power formations should be resisted next. We do not dictate, in terms of the questions Habermas links to ethics, who a person or community 'are' or 'would like to be'. In my view, this forms a key part of our ethics of practice. The question of how persons should live is not up to the narrative practitioner; it is up to those persons themselves.

But this is not a case of naïve individualism. We are not even a priori advocates of the 'human rights' Devri refers to. Human rights discourses – like any other – have their own effects of power, and we remain questioning of these too. For example, such a discourse can be used to support freedom of speech. But when does free speech become gossip, or hate speech? I have witnessed people in powerful institutional positions invoking notions of their 'right to speak', but in ways that silence and intimidate those in less influential positions. Not only do human rights discourses serve a policing function, but the complex and unpredictable ways in which they are deployed signal to us that we cannot even use them to normatively ground the positions we take. We have commitments, but as I see it they lie on a different plain.

Rather, my view is that we are in the business of promoting what Falzon (1998) terms a 'dialogue of forces' (p. 43). This entails a commitment to the task of facilitating the dynamism rather than the fixing of power, the dialogical rather than the monological possibilities of power, so that people are always able to find different ways of being; so that there are always escape routes from specific forms of constraint, control, and constitution. This is an interminable task, such that 'we always have something to do' (Foucault, 1997c, p. 256). Foucault calls this a stance of 'hyper- and pessimistic activism' (p. 256). We cannot adopt a normative stand, consisting in the claim that the person should live according to these standards, these norms, these values, because it is precisely the valorization of social standards, norms, and values that limits the fluidity, flexibility, and dynamism of power relations. We take sides not because we have an a priori commitment to this or that cause, this or that way of being, but, ultimately, because the failure to take sides contributes to the crystallization of power, and to the closing down of escape routes for persons who wish to move away from their particular forms of constitution. In the end, maybe this is a kind of norm; a meta-norm, perhaps. But it is one that, paradoxically, counters any tendency we might have to impose our images of life on the people who consult us.

Second, Habermas' challenge rests on the unwitting assumption that the role of the theorist is to govern, to control, by deciding on how legitimate and illegitimate conduct are to be distinguished. His own proposal is that consensual rationality is the route to such normative determinations. But for Foucault, the elevation of some discourse (such as science or psychoanalysis) to a higher status than others (e.g., local knowledges) – which is essentially what Habermas says should be clarified by rational means – is to promote a certain mode of social control and governance (e.g., about who can speak with authority and who cannot). This is what Foucault wants to avoid, as does the narrative therapist. So, unlike Habermas, we can put forward no system which enables us to declare one kind of power, and hence one kind of resistance, better than another. Such a division would introduce a normative element to our work, leading us to promote various social alignments, norms and values, to prescribe and valorize activities and people associated with the 'good' discourse, while we exclude, punish, or seek to rehabilitate perpetrators of the 'bad' discourse. This is therapy as 'social control' (Hare-Mustin, 1994, p. 20). Instead, Foucault wants to leave this decision – about what to resist and what to support – to local communities and persons living in their own particular circumstances of power. And in large measure, this is what we seek to do as narrative therapists; not to govern our clients by designating their resistances valid or invalid, their ideas rational or irrational, their practices normal or abnormal, but to support them in the life courses they want to pursue and the resistances involved in that process. This, I suspect, is a good way to make power more 'dialogical' in its operations.

We have theoretical grounds, in other words, to not decide in advance which resistances are legitimate and which are not. This is all well and good, but alas we are no closer to understanding why the person resists in the first place. All we know at this stage is that they can, that they sometimes do, and that we cannot make a priori judgements regarding the legitimacy of their resistances. We know that resistance is enabled by the fact that power is not always fully successful, but equally that power's failure, in itself, does not necessarily lead to resistance. Perhaps, then, this failure needs to be accompanied by something like a set of discursive lures enticing us over to different ways of thinking and being. But that idea too has its limitations.

Relying on discursive lures positions the person as docile

This formulation – incorporating the idea that a range of discourses, other than those to which we have become subject, can lure us into their knowledges and practices and thereby provide us with a range of new ways of knowing and being – is an improvement on the assumption that we will resist power simply because we can; because there are times in the fractures of power when our thoughts or actions go unmonitored.

But even so, the notion of the luring, seductive discourse is not enough to account for resistance. This view still retains elements of the social determinism that critics see in the work of Foucault. If we think again of Devri's situation, this account essentially reduces her intentions, and her hopes and dreams for her life – crucial aspects of her experience for the narrative therapist (White, 2007) – to the vagaries and persuasive powers of discourse; to the dynamic relationship between the network of discourses and power dynamics in which her life is played out. We are left with a picture in which it is not Devri herself but new narratives and promised positions that somehow draw her away from a tolerance of her abused position. What will happen next in her life? Well, on such an account we will have to wait for the response of the previously dominant discursive system: what will her husband do, and what impact will this have on her? Will she feel some lingering shame, as the original discourse prescribes? What about familial responses? In other words, which discourse will put forward the most effective lures? The answer to such questions is not determined by Devri herself – indeed, one wonders how, on the constitutionalist account, she could have any role to play at all – but by how well and how firmly she is recruited into the discourse of human rights as it interacts with discourses and practices of family honour, loyalty, the sacredness of marriage, the dictates of culture and religion, and so on. From a thoroughly social perspective, Devri has no *individual* power in the situation, and so her resistance or compliance will be determined, if not by discourse, then at least by discourse dynamics.

It is certainly true that discourse dynamics play a powerful role in influencing our conduct, even our hopes and dreams. This, I think, is one of the main reasons why practices such as re-authoring, re-membering, and outsider-witnessing are so important in narrative therapy. They construct so many thickened lures – communally supported subject positions, preferred interactions, personally resonant ideas and values, historically salient rationales – for the person's preferred ways of being, that they facilitate the building of effective resistances against the resurgent, recuperative, recapturing powers of the problem constituting discourse. But if these practices serve to thicken the individual's preferred position (e.g., human rights versus docile wife), what is the status of *that preference*? Is it determined merely by discourse dynamics, by the competing lures of discourse, and other social forces? It seems to me that we are still left with an understanding of persons as 'no more than wind' (in Veyne, p. 97): an account that, despite their advocacy of a social constitutionalist perspective, neither Foucault nor White would find satisfactory.

Does resistance really require social models?

Evidently, Foucault was uncomfortable committing to a purely social view of the origins of resistance. Somehow it couldn't convincingly overcome the 'wind' problem. Norris (1994) describes how awkward it must have been for him to have so strongly promoted a social constitutionalist perspective on the one hand, while simultaneously advocating 'a strongly oppositional or counter-hegemonic stance' for constituted subjects on the other (p. 166). These two positions do not sit easily together without some significant work on our part. It is in the context of this tension that it might be useful to reflect on Foucault's assertion that resistance does not originate in the individual, but in the social models available to him or her; or in Michael White's words, in the 'materials lying about in society' (2004, p. 103).

But we cannot know how sure Foucault was about this. Hoy (2004) hints that the social models requirement is the unintended corner into which Foucault's constitutionalist, social ontological position had taken him. He was reluctant to concede that the individual himself or herself could have a pre-discursive, pre-social role to play in resistance. Such a concession, says Hoy, might threaten to unravel the whole power/knowledge picture he had spent decades building. But it must have seemed to Foucault that something was not quite right. He seemed to be crediting the human being with nothing more than a capacity to be a servant of discourse.

I wish to remind the reader (and myself) that I am not testing or defending Foucault here. Our overall objective is not to see if Foucault – the author – offers us a coherent picture of the human being, but to ask whether it is possible to build up a coherent picture that takes into account his power/knowledge formulations – the constitutionalist side – with our own therapeutic commitment to some notion of personal agency. So at this stage, we are interrogating not Foucault so much as the constitutionalist perspective that is often associated with him, and its implications for the field of narrative therapy. And so I should repeat that the constitutionalist position is an extreme and only partial interpretation of Foucault's overall work. Nevertheless, if we follow the constitutionalist path all the way to its limits (remembering always that it is not the only pathway Foucault explored), we encounter the idea – as Rorty reads Foucault (Norris, 1994) – that the individual human being is little more than a kind of tabula rasa, an empty void, waiting to be inscribed by social, cultural, and historical forces. And in some ways, Foucault's own work makes this an easy case to make. Against the humanist vision of the sovereign, self-determined, self-authoring being who pre-exists sociality, Foucault responds, early on in his career, that the breaking down of societal discursive and power structures would lead 'man' to be 'erased, like a face drawn in sand at the edge of the sea' (Foucault, 1966, p. 422). In other words, if we lost the social practices that make up the forces of social constitution, the ways of knowing and power relations that give us our 'selves', we human beings would not be left to contemplate this troubling development, or to begin to rebuild a social universe under the steam of our self-sovereignty, as the humanist might suppose. Instead, we would simply vanish into nothingness. The individual is quite literally *nothing* without sociality.

But then why was Foucault 'horrified' by such a social determinist reading of his work? And what led his friend and fellow scholar, Paul Veyne (2010), to characterize such interpretations as 'ridiculous' (p. 97)? Why did Foucault himself continually insist on 'the freedom of individuals', and refuse to see the person as 'no more than wind'? (Veyne, 2010, p. 96). Something is not quite right. And yet Foucault's social models requirement for the appearance of resistance – a position he took, incidentally, not at the beginning of his career, but towards its end – does nothing to change this extreme impression.

I want to suggest that this awkward insistence on the social origins of resistance rests on a conflation, by Foucault, and later by White, of two aspects of resistance. In his discussion of agency in narrative practice in theological settings, Lee (2004) usefully distinguishes between the negative and positive contents of agency. He offers a description of positive agency as the 'intentional movement toward preferred goals', and of negative agency as the 'movement away from or out of subjugating discourses' (p. 226). This struck me not only as a promising way of thinking about agency, and of course resistance, but also as a way out of the social constitutionalist corner we risk painting ourselves into. Inspired by Lee's distinction, I started thinking about resistance in terms of these two elements: a positive and a negative; or rather, an affirmation and a negation. So here is my proposal: the insistence on social models for the emergence of resistance, as per White and Foucault's most explicit writings, refers to the *affirmation* of a particular discourse and its social models, but overlooks or downplays the person's *negation* of, his or her movement away from, problem-saturated stories and practices. We conflate the 'no' with its story, and stories are always social. But what about the 'no'? We will consider that question in the next chapter.

I have found this conceptual opening-up of resistance to be enormously helpful in bringing the agentive individual back into the scene of power relations and discursive practices. So let us at last turn to consider the individual as agent.

5
Embodied Resistance

The constitutionalist perspective that is often associated with Foucault's work, and carried into narrative therapy theorizing via White (e.g., 2004), Epston (e.g., 1993), Madigan (e.g., 2003), and others, is being increasingly developed by Foucauldian scholars in ways that have the potential to move us decisively away from the lingering sense of human docility we might still be carrying at this point. In this chapter, I will use these developments, together with some interpretations of Nietzsche's work, to bring the person's inherent agentive capacities to the fore, in the hope of building an account that might be useful for the narrative practitioner.

We should remember that Foucault oriented to a particular question; and this frames the answers we have been arriving at in the previous chapters. With respect to the relationship between the human subject and the constitutive network of fields of power/knowledge, Foucault's primary question was: what kinds of subjects are produced in power/knowledge? This question flows inevitably from his methodological decision to set aside any presumption of a self-governing, agentive human subject (as he wrote under the pseudonym of Florence, 1998). As Allen (2000) put it:

> Foucault's aim is not to get rid of the concept of subjectivity altogether; instead he sets aside any conception of the subject as constituent in order that he might better understand how the subject is constituted in this particular cultural and historical milieu. (p. 122)

Foucault's original intention was not to *deny* the idea of the active human being, but to omit it from his thought in order to understand the neglected, dimly perceived forces that flow in the other direction. The reasoning, I believe, is solid: any assumptions about such a constituent figure would surely blind us to the force relations that move into his or her life. For instance, if we make the very assumption that Foucault refused to make – that the person is able to act in self-determined, individualistic ways – then it becomes much harder to see the impact of those societal discourses and practices that promote, precisely, self-determination and individualism. It might seem, then, that persons' individualistic intentions, orientations, and conduct arise not from specific sociocultural or historical factors, but from those persons themselves. And to the extent that self-contained individualism comes to seem a natural, innate feature of our existence, we might then assume that we create our own lots in life. It might be reasonable, then, to say that the person trapped in an abusive situation, the person who is labelled in derogatory ways, the individuals who make up segregated and disadvantaged communities, are to be held responsible for their plights. After all, it would seem that we make our own worlds. At the end of the day, such reasoning easily builds into a naïve form of humanism, with the constituent, reality-shaping, meaning-giving individual placed at the centre of human activity.

So, wanting to understand how things work the other way round – how society impacts on our bodies, our thought, our actions – Foucault decided to leave to one side any such assumption. It seems to me that Foucault inadvertently left himself with an image of a derivative, secondary, and hence docile subject, not because he believed this, but because his methodological decision had written out any other possibility. At any rate, somehow, his stance edged from the methodologically disciplined decision to make no assumptions about who is behind the discourse, to the idea (sometimes, but not always expressed) that there is nobody there at all.

While this approach – the suspension of assumptions about the human being in order to understand how power/knowledge produces its subjects – has certainly been invaluable in highlighting the social forces that constitute the person, we might ponder another interesting facet of that Foucauldian strategy; one that brings us to the individual, but now from a different angle; not from the starting point of the sovereign humanist subject and then working outwards towards the social, but from the perspective of societal power and discourse dynamics and working back to its preconditions. Thinking about it this way, we come to a question which Foucault addressed only implicitly: what sort of human being is *presupposed or required* in order for power/knowledge fields to function?

As Deleuze (1990) has hinted, Foucault could not have seriously posed this question before working out significant aspects of his power/knowledge formulation. Perhaps we ask too much to expect him to have fully answered it. It has thus been left to subsequent scholars to open up spaces for the consideration of this and related questions. So now we can wonder: if power/knowledge works in this way or that, has this or that effect on us, does that tell us anything about who we are? Or, we can adapt the question critical realist Roy Bhaskar (2008) asks ('what must be the case for science to be possible', p. 29): what must the person be like for power/knowledge to work? If we are to think of power/knowledge as a factory that produces human identities, of what kinds of raw materials should its subjects be composed? And then: if we were somehow other than what we are, would power/knowledge still work? Would it have to work differently?

Variations of such questions have been tackled – albeit not in so many words – by numerous authors (e.g., Falzon, 1993, 1998; Gordon, 1999; O'Leary, 2002). In addition, others, closer to Foucault (Deleuze, 1988; Veyne, 2010), remind us that Foucault is a Nietzschean, and as such built his analyses of power on certain (though seldom articulated) presumptions about the human being. Together, these explorations suggest that the Foucauldian subject is a far more active figure than his constitutionalist position (the one we have incorporated into our narrative work) allows, and far more alive and powerful than his critics claim. Perhaps, also, these developments can help us make sense of those interviews, lectures, and other statements in which Foucault insists on a creative, self-directing, even 'free' human subject as power's condition of possibility (e.g., 1982, p. 221). We can understand such comments, which, to borrow a phrase from White (2007), seem 'out of phase' (p. 61) with Foucault's constitutionalist work on power/knowledge, without thinking that he thereby gave up on the latter and collapsed into a humanistic perspective. Rather, we retain our vision of the considerable forces of social constitution, but now as acting not on a passive, docile body, but on an 'active body' (Foucault, 1977, p. 137): a living, agentive, embodied being invested in his or her own freedom.

I would like to put forward three proposals that have arisen for me following my engagement with this post-Foucault Foucauldian thought. First, power can only work if its subjects are already prediscursive, embodied, and active beings, corporeally endowed with their own capacities and energies. Second, the energies and actions of this embodied being resist, exceed, and overflow the impositions of power. And third, in order to avoid being dissolved into chaos, meaninglessness, and nothingness, the person must direct these resistances into further, perhaps new, forms of subjection.

Let us examine each proposal in turn.

Power relies on prediscursive, active bodies

The first thing that struck me when I studied this literature was the idea that the power relations Foucault describes can only function if human beings have an inherent, extra-discursive, a priori, and corporeally based capacity to act in the world (e.g., Falzon, 1993; Gordon, 1999; O'Leary, 2002). This reading privileges the 'active body' to which Foucault referred (1977, p. 137), rather than the image he gives elsewhere of the body as docile and malleable as 'formless clay' (p. 135). The clay metaphor only superficially coheres with the idea of power's shaping of identity (as we discussed in Chapter 2), and does not tally with Foucault's talk of the body's inherent capacities and forces, nor with his insistence on freedom as a condition of possibility for power's operations (c.f., Falzon, 1993). Rather, power requires not only the pre-existence of a particular 'raw material' – the body – but needs it also to be already alive, active, moving, energized, and capable of learning to conduct itself in self-directed, though ultimately discursively prescribed ways. This thesis immediately suggests that power does not 'produce' us in the radical sense of bringing us into existence, and undermines any claim that there is nothing at all beneath or behind the story.

Before exploring this proposal in more depth, it should be acknowledged that talk of an actual material body – with capacities that exceed those of a lump of clay – is surprisingly contentious in the context of post-structural, Foucauldian literature, which has tended to emphasize the body as a kind of 'writing pad' (Kirby, 1991, p. 13) on which discourse, ably assisted by power, inscribes its messages and requirements. I will refer to this as Foucault's inscription approach. Foucault was not so much interested in building a scheme for understanding the body itself, and limited (for the most part) his focus to the question of how power shapes, acts on, and makes use of it (Dreyfus and Rabinow, 1982). We have seen power working this way in earlier discussions on the constituted subject: consider Petra's production as a romantic subject, based on her subjection as an embodied woman; or Oscar's production as a weak man, based on the cultural meanings attached to male bodies and their masculinity; or Nobisa's shame around her pregnancy, built on prevailing cultural expectations about how young, unmarried women should conduct their bodies. In the inscription approach, the body – its appearance, its shape, its movements, gestures, and performances – is best seen not as a pre-existing material entity with its own energies and forces, but solely as a product of particular historical, cultural, and discursive circumstances. Indeed, it is credited with no active role to play in power, other than to be its endlessly malleable raw material, much like clay, ready to be sculpted into whatever forms power requires. On this account, the body is not a force in its own right, and so it has no means of interacting with power except through total compliance and docility.

There is a danger in incorporating into our understanding of inscription a parallel view of the body as simultaneously a pre-existing living set of forces – as I will do here. Any definitive claim about the prediscursive body would make us vulnerable to being branded 'essentialist' (Kirby, 1991, p. 4). For instance, if we were to suggest something like, 'prior to its exposure to power and discourse, the body is, already, in reality, this, and not that', we might be tempted to distinguish between 'natural, normal' bodies and bodily conduct (those that line up with our definition) and 'unnatural, abnormal' bodies and their conduct (those that do not). From that point it becomes possible to form and legitimize oppressive and controlling normative judgements about how persons should and should not conduct their bodies, and hence their actions, in the social spaces of their lives. Essentialism might also lead, as we have already seen in cases discussed in earlier chapters, to the attachment of certain socially constructed identities to particular bodies, along dimensions of gender, race, body size and shape, and so on. Kirby (1991) has noted, with reference to debates in feminism, that the fear of essentialism is so great that many refuse to even recognize the body as a material presence at all, preferring to locate it squarely within the realm of discourse and social practice. But, she suggests, the act of denying 'embodied existence' is surely 'a nonsense' (1991, p. 17), and Foucault would no doubt have agreed (e.g., 1977, p. 138). Indeed, Falzon (1993) argues that Foucault's work could not be understood without, precisely, this materially existing body, which precedes power and is, therefore, not merely its product, as the extreme inscription approach suggests. Nevertheless, the point is that we will need to be careful in how we talk about embodied existence, and remain cognizant of the question: does talk about a prediscursive, active body entail a reversion to an essentialist account? I will engage more fully with this question at the end of the second proposal (below), once we have said enough about the body to consider it more carefully.

So, what is the significance of this talk of bodies? There are three points that arise for me here. First, we should note that for Foucault the individual is nothing more than the body and its conduct, and it is out of the meanings inscribed by cultural discourse on, precisely, the body and its conduct that an identity or sense of self emerges. As in Nietzsche, the 'self' is seen to emerge from the body. It is our existence as physical, embodied beings who take up space and act in the world that enables us to take up (culturally specific) subject positions in the first place (Falzon, 1993). Indeed, we become subjects only to the extent that our *'material bodies...* come into contact with operations of power' (Ryan, 2012, p. 16, emphasis added).

Second, Falzon (1993) sees in Foucault's depiction of the body a guarantee that we – our bodies and our identities – will always be grounded in the particular sociocultural and historical worlds and eras in which we live. This grounding precludes any possibility of a transcendental, ahistorical, or decontextualized understanding of who we are. Falzon (1993) contrasts Foucault's view with the humanist position, which we will remember is the stance against which much of Foucault's work develops. Humanism, says Falzon, creates an image of a sovereign and disembodied human being, who is able to transcend the particular world in which he or she lives, to lift himself or herself out of contemporary social conditions. Falzon argues that the Foucauldian view of the embodied human being – whose embodiment insures his or her grounding within the world of specific social powers, activities, and historical conditions – shows up the humanist account as inhuman and abstract. Humanism, in fact, tears the person out of the actual concrete world in which he or she lives. There can be, says Falzon, no 'ghostly authorial subject "behind" our acts, removed from concrete human existence' (1993, p. 2). How can such an abstract, disembodied figure be effected by, or have an effect on, the real world? On the Foucauldian account, we are not 'ghostly authors' – invisible minds or souls driving our bodily activities from behind the scenes – but only concrete, material beings. This means not only that any escape from power relations is impossible, but also that, and as a consequence, we have no choice but to develop our identities – our subject positions – in historically, culturally, and socially specific ways.

And third, for Falzon, discourse and power do not 'produce' the body in a literal sense, but rely on its prior presence as an energized, moving, already living raw material. Clearly, Falzon sees in Foucault's work not only the inscribed body, as emphasized in *Discipline and Punish* (1977) and many other works, but also a living, potentially agentive one. In fact, says Falzon, 'it is the corporeal, active human being, and *not power*, which is fundamental to Foucault's account' (p. 8, emphasis added). The body is the primary, 'basic' factor, and stands as the concrete underpinning of and precondition for the social forces of power, which are only 'secondary and derivative' (Falzon, 1993, p. 9).

To develop this idea of the 'living body', let us consider elements of the relationship between bodily activity on the one hand, and the social power dynamics into which these activities may be recruited on the other. Our bodies are extraordinarily active, and are constantly engaged in some kind of movement. We itch, scratch, slump, get up, look around; we orient to sensory stimulation; we breathe in and out, and our chests and shoulders move accordingly; we close and open our eyes; we move our fingers, arms, and legs to facilitate sleep, or for no particular reason; our faces move in all manner of ways, without any discursive prescriptions. Now, many of these voluntary as well as involuntary movements will be recruited into – or inscribed on by – social power dynamics. As Falzon has highlighted, it is precisely the possibility of the recruitment of the active body that allows disciplinary power to function. Our corporeally based potential for activity and movement makes us excellent candidates for subjection: my slowed movements, my tired eyes, my yawn, might be taken up by a friend (or indeed by my therapist or my client) as boredom, and lead to an array of moves and countermoves, interpretations, and counter-interpretations. I remember how, as a seven-year-old boy, my slumped shoulders – of which I was entirely unaware – were interpreted by one of my teachers as 'a lack of self-confidence'. Because I exist in fields of power, I cannot control the ways in which my body, my movements, and my occupation of space, will be taken up by others; I cannot determine the manner of my recruitment. When I involuntarily move my arms while asleep, I might bump into my wife who in turn interprets this as my unexpressed hostility towards her because of an argument we had earlier. Before I know it, my involuntary movement has me in the middle of a power dynamic. So our movements can be captured and invested (or inscribed) with culturally and socially specific meanings. But for this to occur, these bodily movements must necessarily pre-exist their discursive capture, or there would be nothing for discourse to grasp.

While we can say that our bodies' active movements are often interpreted and given discursive significance, and thereby entered into a field of power relations, we should not be confused into concluding that this field of power relations *produced* this or that movement. Yes, power and discourse inscribe, but they surely cannot inscribe the entire universe into existence. We surely ask too much of discourse if we expect it to serve as the original authorial cause of my tired eyes, my sleep movements, my itching ankle and the scratch I use to ease it. All discourse can do is effect what Nealon (2008) calls a fine-'tuning' (p. 106) of my pre-existing corporeal aliveness, my bodily movements, by recruiting me and others to deploy the concepts and interpretations it provides. Thus, my wife might invoke discourses of unconscious hostility (she is, after all, a psychologist) and thereby usher in a field of conflict regarding my motivations for bumping her in the night; I might (or might not) wonder if I was indeed angry with her, and vow to address the issues so that I don't further disturb her sleep. The discourse of unconscious hostility might in such ways fine-tune my movement by giving it a particular meaning, urging me to fix the problems it represents, and thereby to alter the movement itself (e.g., so I no longer bump into her). But I think we ask too much of this discourse, even with the significant support it gains from multiple aligned social practices, to ask that it take full responsibility for the movement itself. Similarly, my schoolteacher deploys a discourse of body language, claiming my posture and giving it a meaning that went on to influence the way I carried myself, as well as my thoughts about how I came across to others. But can we be sure that my slumped shoulders as a seven-year-old were a discursive product?

And this, I think, is what Falzon is saying is important to recognize in the Foucauldian perspective. Power does not produce the living body, but orchestrates its pre-existing energies and movements to make it more useful to the particular society in which it finds itself. The living body comes first. Power then influences what shape it will assume, and invests it with particular subjectivities, identities, or senses of self. We are also interpellated in the process, and so we come to participate in the discursive shaping of our bodies and their conduct.

So, if power/knowledge works, for instance, to produce Oscar in its own terms in the form 'failed man', then this operation rests on his capacity to act accordingly; to organize his body movements in the proper way (e.g., his tendency to avoid eye contact, to look downwards, to slump his shoulders), to experience himself more generally as a failed man, and to perform this role in the social domain. Or perhaps, because this is not a deterministic business, he strives to present a counter-image of himself, again within the same discourse, to carry his body in more 'manly ways'. Similarly, the success of Devri's positioning as a docile woman in an abusive relationship will depend on her capacity to enact precisely that position: to regulate her voice and still it when necessary, to carry her body in religiously and culturally approved ways when in the company of other women and men (e.g., not to be too expansive or 'masculine' in her movements), to dress in certain ways, and so on.

The prediscursive aliveness of the body is brought out even more clearly by O'Leary (2002), who refers to this bodily being as the 'human animal' (p. 118); the earthly, corporeal base that Foucault presupposes, and without which his postulated power/knowledge network could not operate. In other words, we should not confuse 'power over' persons with those persons' 'power to' do what is expected of them (Patton, 1989, p. 268). Similarly, Nealon (2008, p. 104) says that power asks two kinds of questions pertaining to its subjects. The first is 'What can it be?' That is, can Oscar be made into a masculinized subject, Petra a romantic, and Devri a religiously devout and honourable wife? Can these persons be fashioned into the kinds of objects that power requires for its purposes? But the second question is: 'What can it do?' What can these persons *already* do, which power can then seize and fashion to its own ends? In answer to this last question, we are referred to the notion of the human animal, with its energies, capacities, and forces.

Let us recall Alphonso Lingis' (1977) reading of the Nietzschean position: 'There are no longer … any persons … only interpretations and interpretations of interpretations' (p. 42). Well, we might not call this human animal with its raw capacities a 'person', and O'Leary (2002) maintains that it is not yet a 'subject', not yet a product of discourse (p. 118). But there is at least *something* alive lurking beneath the interpretation. At least, then, we are not simply dead things, mannequins, being moved around by discourse and power; at minimum, we are beings with our own 'animal' capacities, movements, powers, forces, and energies. There is *something* – some bare minimum 'material' (O'Leary, 2002, p. 118) – which exists and lives prior to our subjectivity.

While this something is not yet a subject, not yet socially constructed or discursively formed, I will argue that it does *matter* for our understanding of the human capacity for agency and resistance. We should not discount this possibility simply because it is not a product of discourse or social practice, in contrast to virtually everything else we think and talk about in narrative practice. Coming close to the dangers of an essentialist position (to which we will not succumb, as I will argue below), we can say that this human animal is a kind of a priori figure, insofar as it exists prior to discourse and power; it precedes the forces that constitute our identities.

In sum, the Foucauldian notion of the subject as both a product and vehicle of power requires us to have at least two interrelated properties: we must be embodied, with animal energies and capacities, and we must be able to fine-tune these capacities so that we can be put to use, and play a part in social activities in a particular location, culture, and set of social circumstances. Already this means that we need to revise our vision of the human being as nothing but interpretation, as made up of nothing but stories and stories of stories.

The question then becomes: does this living embodied being have some kind of 'directionality'? Is it just a bundle of energy, a workhorse waiting for direction? Or does it have some kind of 'inbuilt' directional tendency – in the way that Freud's subject tends towards pleasure over pain, Rogers' towards self-actualization, and Beck's towards rational appraisals? This is an important question, and any answer in the affirmative would require us to clarify the post-structural status of this formulation, so that we do not edge down the path towards essentialism. Nevertheless, I propose that there is something that the human animal is prone to doing: resist. Resistance, I suggest, far from being only a product of social dynamics, is grounded in our very corporeality.

The body resists power

My second proposal, which builds on the first, is this: the capacity for resistance is immanent in the body, and precedes the person's subjection in discourse. On the one hand, this is at odds with Foucault's and White's explicit stance that social models and discourses are required for the emergence of resistance, as we saw in the previous chapter. And yet, on the other hand, Foucault's references to the 'freedom' of individuals (e.g., 1982, p. 221; 1997d, p. 293) and the living body as the very condition of power's operations seems to suggest a capacity for resistance that inheres in the body (Falzon, 1993). Furthermore, at other points he indicates that the rejection of a particular course of action (or position or strategy) does not require the presence of alternatives (e.g., Foucault, 2000b). On this latter account, the person can refuse without justification, without a social model to support such refusal, and without a plan B. The human capacity for refusal is seen to precede his or her exposure to social practices and narratives: this part of us precedes power. This way of reading Foucault's work is supported by Zivkovic and Hogan (2008), who indicate that 'resistance is the "always already" of power; resistance precedes power' (p. 190). Clearer still is Deleuze's (1988) summary of Foucault's position: 'The final word on power is that resistance *comes first*' (p. 74, emphasis added).

But what does it mean to say that resistance 'comes first'? We can discern two complementary, rather than mutually contradictory, ways of thinking about this, which relate to the two orientations to the body referred to above – the inscription approach and the living body approach – and which I, following Lee (2004), will refer to as the positive and negative aspects of resistance, respectively.

Positive resistance

On the one hand, we can offer a 'positive' account of resistance. This is a more or less storied resistance, with its own positive (i.e., present, existing) meanings or contents. This is the only position allowed by the thoroughgoing constitutionalist perspective, and corresponds, as I see it, with the view of the body (and its conduct) as no more than a surface inscribed by discourse. The argument here would be that resistance comes first because it comes from other, alternative discourses and practices, which are already there in our social networks, waiting to recruit and make their mark on us (and which we described in the previous chapter in terms of their 'lures'). We assume that because we live in a discursive multiverse, in which various discourses exert some kind of shaping or constitutive force on us, we are always simultaneously pulled in different directions. The more complex our social worlds become (i.e., the more diverse our social discourses, and hence personal narratives), the more discursive tensions there will be for us to negotiate. In one sense, then, to claim that resistance precedes power is to say that from the perspective of any particular 'dominant' discourse (e.g., masculinity, romance, or gendered submission), numerous other discourses will always already be at hand to promote resistance against the former's attempts to render us its subjects.

For example, Devri – who was caught up in an abusive relationship, and found in the idea of human rights a way of justifying and thickening her resistance (see Chapter 4) – might at some level already have been recruited into something like, something approximating, or something with useful ingredients of, a human rights discourse, long before meeting her husband. And so when, later on, the paternalistic discourse of male control over female partners becomes a reality in her life, the already available discourses – ideas, practices, values – that are susceptible of investment into the notion of human rights, can be seen to have already equipped Devri with the capacity to resist. Re-authoring practices would not be possible without some such elements in her personal history; without – to think of this in terms of her embodiment – her having been in some sense 'marked' or subjectified in her own history by practices related to something like human rights discourse. In this sense, re-authoring requires that resistance comes first. Thus, Devri and I were able to identify moments from various points in her life in which she demonstrated a valuing of certain things that linked up with the notion of human rights. For instance, she described how appalled she was as a child that a particular individual at her school had shown 'absolutely no respect for the next person'. The re-emergence of such knowledges, performative know-how, and the resistances they enable, might be delayed for various reasons: she falls in love, she follows family tradition, and then when troubles emerge she must deal with the cultural taboo on divorce, and so on. But we can say, nevertheless, that this resistance – which is not quite 'hers', but which she can utilize to the extent that she has become in some manner subject to human rights discourse – 'comes first' in the sense that she is thereby to some degree experientially and, hence, corporeally (behaviourally and with a bodily sense) equipped to resist practices that subvert values and ideas associated with human rights.

Such a positive account of resistance – seeing resistance as already having some of its own discursive contents; in this case something to do with human rights and respecting others – construes it as preceding a *particular discourse; but not discourse per se*. This resistance is still a discursive product. While this view is entirely consistent with the constitutionalist aspects of power I have tried to articulate, Lee (2004) maintains that narrative therapists tend to limit themselves by attending only to such a positive, content-filled account of agency (or in this case, resistance). It does not exhaust the matter. The typically neglected negative aspect of resistance offers us a small but significant addition to this account.

Negative resistance

Negative resistance can be seen as the embodied refusal which precedes not only a *particular* discourse, but discourse as such. It is negative in the sense that it entails a refusal of a current identity, but since it lacks its own narrative or discursive contents, it cannot yet affirm what the person should become. It is a bodily resistance, not yet a discursive one.

Many see this notion of the body as a resisting force as implicit in Foucault's work. For example, Judith Butler (1989) notes that Foucault sometimes describes the body as if it were 'a prediscursive multiplicity of bodily forces' that 'disrupt the regulating practices of cultural coherence imposed upon that body by a regulatory regime' (p. 607). She sees this as inconsistent with his more prevalent approach to the body as inscribed by power. However, others consider the theses of inscription and the living, resisting body to be complementary rather than mutually exclusive understandings. Falzon (1993), for instance, sees the 'irreducibly resistant' body as key to understanding power's always incomplete hold over the human being (p. 10). We have also encountered O'Leary's (2002) belief that what he calls the 'human animal' stands as a precondition for Foucault's understanding of power; an animal, he goes on to say, comprised of a 'brute, disorganized and relatively chaotic set of capacities, powers and forces' (p. 118). Resistance is inevitable here, as chaotic 'animal' forces will always, by definition, threaten to disrupt discursively imposed order. Also on this theme, Veyne (2010) maintains that Foucault shares with Nietzsche the view that '(e)very individual is a centre of energy that...is never neutralized or abolished' (pp. 96–97); a centre of energy, in other words, that power can never completely tame. And, finally, Deleuze (1988) sees Foucault's notion of 'man as a living being' (Foucault, 1990a, p. 144) as involving a resistance embedded in life itself.

> Life becomes resistance to power when power takes life as its object...resistance becomes the power of life, a vital power that cannot be contained within the paths of a particular diagram. Is not...a certain vitalism, in which Foucault's thought culminates? Is not life this capacity to resist force? And for Foucault as much as for Nietzsche, it is in man himself that we must look for the set of forces and functions which resist the death of man...(For Foucault) there is no telling what man might achieve 'as a living being', as the set of forces that resist.
>
> (Deleuze, 1988, p. 77)

I will try to thicken this view of the embodied human being as a set of forces that resists by extending the first assumption I made above (the active body) with a second, decidedly Nietzschean – and perhaps, as have seen, implicitly Foucauldian – one: the body is not a singular, coherent physical object, possessing universal drives or needs, but 'a multiple phenomenon' composed of 'irreducible forces' (Deleuze, 2006, p. 37). As O'Leary (2002) suggests, these diverse and unpredictable forces do not of their own accord (i.e., in the absence of social power dynamics) cohere or orchestrate in some universal manner that we might think of as 'essential'. For example, the body's forces are not universally organized around a pleasure principle, a drive for survival or reproduction, a directed urge to satiate particular instinctual needs and drives, or any other such essential or singular activity. Instead, as an inherently diverse and 'multiple phenomenon' the body must be, in itself, nothing-in-particular. It does not have a 'determinate character' (Falzon, 1993, p. 3). But it is precisely this multiplicity – not its supposed 'docility' – that makes the body a suitable object for the operations of power. That is, the body's multiplicity lends it a quality of malleable plasticity, making it pliable enough to be shaped into the discursive forms society prescribes for it.

In the context of these two assumptions (the body as living body, and as a multiplicity of forces which resists), we are led to what might seem like a rather obvious point, but which nevertheless is worth making: the body is not discourse, and discourse is not the body. Or as Butler (1989) put it, reading between the lines of Foucault's writings, 'history is "inscribed" or "imprinted" onto a body that is not history' (p. 607). We have seen that others make a similar point (e.g., Deleuze, 1988; Falzon, 1993; Veyne, 2010). There are, in other words, important though typically unstated differences between these two objects of our concern. While the body is composed of multiple, diverse, discontinuous, decentred, and dispersed energies and forces – which some call 'chaos' (Heidegger, 1987; O'Leary, 2002) – discourse has a tendency towards order, continuity, coherence, and, ultimately, centredness (Laclau and Mouffe, 2001). Yes, it is true that in postmodern thought we consider meaning to be always 'slippery', uncertain, and deferred. But this slipperiness is not in the essence of discourse itself, nor is it prescribed by it. Instead, it arises out of discourse's relative failure or slippage in the course of its interaction with multiple other discourses. In a sense, meaning changes when other discourses intervene. Its slipperiness points us to the *disruption* of an otherwise ordered, coherent, centring discourse. To the extent that a discourse is bound up with power, and hence successfully produces socially coordinated activity, it moves towards certainty, centredness, and the enclosure of the social fields it describes. Here, we are talking about its enclosure of and imposition on the human body and its conduct. Thus, the reductive order of discourse is imposed on the body's diverse multiplicity, complexity is simplified, and the streaming forces of life are arrested in places where they are captured and enclosed into knowledge categories.

Of course, this is not necessarily a bad thing. As I argued in my earlier discussion of Nietzsche, we need to believe in *something*, and the discipline and order that knowledge provides make it possible to build a life: to capitalize on life experience, to make sense of and address contingent dangers and challenges, to produce and share meaning, to coordinate activities, to live with purpose, even to be part of society. But this nevertheless involves a reduction in complexity: the body becomes a human body (Falk, 1985) – a subjectified body – only to the extent that its multiplicity is sculpted and reduced by discourse, allowing it in turn to be seen and engaged with in the light of socially meaningful interpretation.

The image that emerges here is one of discourse, in its disciplinary effects, curtailing the flow of the body's forces as well as its performative options (even as it shapes some of them into socially recognizable forms). It not only takes the body's chaos and lends it order, but in doing so grants it what Foucault (1977) called a 'soul' – an enduring and deeply felt sense of one's self, in the form of a constituted subject – which becomes 'the prison of the body' (p. 30). That is, the constituted subject operates as a kind of principle that, as we have seen, emerges in the first instance from the manner of the body's discursive inscription or recruitment, before performing its function of governing the body and its multiple movements, gestures, speech, and other actions and modes of expression. It is in this sense that it comes to 'imprison' the body. Such imprisonment can be conceptualized through Klossowski's positing of knowledge's 'principle of conservation' (2005, p. 79): as knowledge or narrative provides us with positions or identities – ways of knowing ourselves – it simultaneously hems us in and prescribes our conduct, thought, and affect. It holds us in the proper place. A similar point is made by Bakhtin (1984), for whom the narrative threatens to convert what he thinks of as the 'unfinalizable' human being into a finalized product: a sutured, enclosed, defined, known once-and-for-all thing.

However, while discipline and subjectification do, in fact, achieve a level of mastery over some of the body's forces, the human being is never finalized or closed off to other possibilities in the process. Foucault's preferred explanation for this seems to be that this is due to the limitations of power itself – a position that we have seen is echoed by White (2004), and which stands as a cornerstone for the constitutionalist, and indeed narrative, account of resistance. But according to the Nietzschean position adopted here, it is the *living body* and its multiple forces, which flow over, around, and through discursive capture, that exceeds the arresting categories discourse tries to impose on it. Resistance is guaranteed – it 'comes first' – to the extent that human beings are always already characterized by the 'excess and overflow of blossoming bodily being' (Nietzsche, 1968, p. 422). For Nietzsche, the body's energies are like a stream whose complexity and multiplicity exceeds or overflows the order society tries to put on it (Heidegger, 1987; Nietzsche, 1968, p. 422). In other words, and to borrow Foucault's metaphor, the body's forces and its conduct inevitably exceed the constraints imposed by its jailer – the self it has come to be.

This body resists then, not because it contains some essential drive, principle, or need which urges the person to challenge unfitting social demands, but by virtue of its excess and overflowing of society's prescriptions. This means, as I suggested above, that the body's malleability – despite the fact that it is precisely this that makes it amenable to being shaped into any number of subject positions – should not be confused for docility. Certainly, the pliable body cannot resist in universal, predictable, or pre-scripted ways. It has no coherent internal 'script' on which to act; no essence on whose behalf resistance is aroused. Consider this against the theoretical case of the pleasure principle in classical psychoanalysis. This is a force which, let us imagine, urges the child to resist society's attempts to recruit him or her into certain impulse control or superego practices. But if we conceive of the body as irreducible multiplicity of forces, it becomes evident that it can have no such stable, internal, enduring, and singular guiding force. Rather, this body resists, not because it is one thing facing up to a society which tells it to be something else – more or less, the essentialist position – but because it is always already *many things* facing up to a society which tells it is *one thing, this thing*: a loser, a schizophrenic, a criminal, a man, a woman.

The product of these multiple bodily forces is an individual who never accepts the forms of subjectivity imposed on him or her in any finalized, permanent sense, a fate which would threaten to obliterate his or her essential, embodied fluid multiplicity. It must, somewhere, somehow, disrupt what it is made into. It is, therefore, *the individual*, rather than only power's limitations, which insures that power's hold is always incomplete, tentative, and provisional. This position is echoed by the French philosopher, Pierre Klossowski, whose book *Nietzsche and the Vicious Circle* was described by Foucault as 'the best book on philosophy…(he had) ever read'. Klossowski (2005) argued that the Nietzschean view of life involves a living organism which, in its multiplicity of internal forces, 'cannot tolerate the state of equilibrium' (p. 81). It is not easily settled, and cannot accept once and for all the limitations imposed on it by discourse and power. Instead, the relationship between the living being and social power dynamics is reflective of a 'principle of disequilibrium' (p. 79), such that when the latter predominates, the former intervenes and exceeds the levels imposed on it. This active intervention insures that power's capture is always provisional, unsteady, off-centre, and incomplete. Again, we have an image of a living, dynamic individual, who is always equipped to unsettle the identity-prescribing hold power seeks to have over him or her.

We sometimes see this resistance in the body's aliveness, in performances of a kind of corporeal excess which defies the limits imposed by discourse. On this account, even as the body accepts the impositions of discipline (which it must, as we shall see in the next section), it proves to be a challenging material to work with. It doesn't sit still, and from early childhood it has to be repeatedly and systematically trained so that its movements are in accord with the form expected of it in the particular sociocultural milieu in which it finds itself. Considerable and ongoing work must be undertaken to train this dynamic, living body to consistently use the right (e.g., culturally or gender-appropriate) physical gestures with the appropriate ranges of movement: the right volume and tone of voice, the correct mouth and tongue movements to facilitate a particular kind of speech, the right amount of eye contact depending on the rules of a particular culture, the right amount of pressure and precision on the page as the body habituates to writing, and so on. Even so – and this is the point – as disciplined subjects we seldom get it 100 per cent right. We overflow our discursive imprisonment in the most banal and unintentional of ways: we cough, sneeze, laugh, or yawn when we're not supposed to; we stumble when we walk, or we move faster, more expansively, and take up more space than we should; we stammer and forget our lines, or we don't stick to the point – we use more words, tell more stories, and speak louder than is expected. Our bodies groan under the weight of discourse and its restrictive, imprisoning disciplinary specifications, and then we inevitably slip out from under it.

Such a slipping-out from under the weight of discourse was apparent in my conversations with Devri about her unbearably controlling home and marital situation. As she became more relaxed in our meetings, I noticed that her bodily movements became more expressive and animated than one might have expected given the prescriptions for a woman's behaviour in her cultural and religious environment. I saw how multiple little movements and gestures of her body troubled and overflowed the story that had been constructed for it. She seemed, quite literally, to exceed the size and shape expected of her movements. Somehow, the stories of her as docile, as somebody's property, could never really fit her body's dynamism, which appeared to struggle against, and disrupt, the positions imposed on her. Furthermore, this resistance is evident not only in the body's spontaneous movements, but also in its more socialized, trained performances, such as in speech. Devri's verbalized objections to being treated as a 'thing', and as her husband's possession, for instance, immediately hints at a languaged overflowing and an unsettling of the docile position into which she had been installed.

Of course, as we saw in the last section, it is possible to conceptualize Devri's resisting movements and verbalizations as grounded in some heretofore and unappreciated self-knowledge concerning human rights, or at least something like it. But as we hear her anger about her abusive situation, and see her more expansive gestures, at a time when the relevance of human rights discourse had not yet occurred to her, why would we insist that it is this as yet unarticulated discourse that invisibly authors her resistance? Why would we grant such prominence to a discourse which, in the moments prior to its elaboration in therapy, was nowhere to be found? After all, the notion of human rights only emerged when it was elicited as a set of responses to certain therapeutic questions, reflected upon, and scaffolded into narrative form in the dialogue. It seems to me rather that Devri (and myself as therapist) seizes on human rights discourse in more opportunistic fashion; not quite because it was *already* meaningful to her, but because she wished to reject her patriarchal, abusive situation, and, following the movement of our conversation, sought a way to make sense of this desire and its consequences. The narrative therapist's way of facilitating such sense making, broadly speaking, is to connect up the person's resistance with his or her values and ethics (see Chapter 7). In the process it may begin to *seem* that human rights was already lurking somewhere in the background of Devri's life. But does it not merely seem this way because it is so fitting in her particular situation – after all, the notion of human rights is linguistically and narratively convenient, an easily available 'opposite' term to that of abuse – and because the values we find resonate with the notion of human rights, in turn making it feel familiar and close to her experience? I wonder, in other words, if human rights discourse works well here, not because it was already there, but because it makes for a good but *retrospective* narrative and experiential fit.

It seems unlikely that a pre-existing human rights discourse motivated Devri's resistance. I believe it is more plausible to think of her overflowing movements and speech in terms of negative resistance; actions which come together to signify a negation or an exceeding of what she has been made into, but not (yet) an affirmation of what she should become: an escape from one enclosure in the stream of her life, but not yet a decisive reaching out for another. It is an enactment of what in words we might think of as 'I must move; I am hemmed in; this

is not what I want; I am more than this', but without the requirement of accompanying alternative stories and sets of subject positions.
Of course, as we shall see in the next section, reaching out for another
meaning or story is necessary for change, but my point is that it is
often a secondary step – an act of narrative construction, or therapeutic
co-construction, to prevent the person's recuperation by the rejected discourse, or a collapse into meaninglessness. It is in this sense that we can
understand Falzon's view that the body and its resistances are primary,
or 'basic', while the interpretative, story-generating work of discourse
and power is 'secondary and derivative' (1993, p. 9). Devri's embodied
resistance comes first, and the story she comes to make of it is secondary.

I want to suggest, furthermore, that the body's inherent capacity for
resistance is not hidden from power. In fact, it seems to me not only
that power recognizes that the individual's resistance is *already there*,
but that it strives – though it is not always successful – to *anticipate*
and be ready to counteract it (c.f., Prozorov, 2007a). We might even
think of psychoanalysis and certain other forms of therapy as enterprises
devoted to the anticipation of resistance, full as they are of interpretive
stories designed to lend pre-scripted meanings to even the most involuntary of actions and movements. But such anticipations apply also to
everyday situations. We – as power's ordinary, though often unwitting
agents – implicitly recognize that there is always something uncertain
about a person's given identity, or location in a constituted position.
And so we are ready to intervene, to remind the person of his or her
duties and responsibilities, of who he or she is supposed to be in this or
that situation, and thereby counter his or her counter-normative moves.
We recognize the change in the divorced man, for example, who has
decided after a few weeks of grieving to go on a date, and we wonder
if this is premature; if he is moving to a place that is not yet properly
'his'. So, armed with good intentions and a powerful discursive system
of 'common sense', we urge him to take it slow, to give it time. We might
not have anticipated precisely these actions, but our socialization, nevertheless, lends us a readiness to counter actions which contradict our
discursively shaped understandings of what is appropriate and normative in any given instance. We *expect* resistance – it is no real surprise –
and are in some measure trained to counter it.

Recall also Oscar's decision to open up to his father about the abuse
he had suffered in his marriage (see Chapter 3). This decision, the honesty and vulnerability of which threatened to undermine the masculine
requirement that Oscar should present himself in 'manly' ways, had the
potential to permit new ways of thinking about his situation. But his

father, unwittingly perhaps, did not allow this miniscule, exploratory movement to develop. Instead, through his judgemental questioning ('how does a man allow that to happen?...'), he managed to pull Oscar back into his constituted position as a failed man. It seems as if Oscar could not be trusted to keep doing what his father (and many in masculinist culture) understood as the right thing to do. His resistance was, in a sense, anticipated.

It seems then that for a constituting discourse to work effectively, it often needs to do much more than stamp the person once with its mark. Instead, it calls on its various vehicles or representatives – persons and communities – to maintain the person in his or her constituted position. Because the person exceeds his or her enclosure in a reductive, simplified, singular space, subject-positioning tends not to be effective as only a singular act or event. Instead, it must be a repeated, ever-present, and often increasingly refined process if it is to hold the person in his or her designated place. Thus, Oscar must be repeatedly reminded of who he is, particularly when he threatens – as he inevitably will – to subvert his designated position. Power must come from everywhere, and *labour* via ongoing coordinated social action, precisely because it knows that the person can and will resist.

This notion of the multiple body, whose forces overflow and imbalance the imprisoning effects of discourse, grants the human being a far more active role in resistance than the strong constitutionalist positions allows, and offers up an optimistic vista for the narrative practitioner. It suggests that the human being would not be doomed to docility – to slavishly reproduce himself or herself in unwanted terms – if there was not available some alternative discourse to the ones that currently describe and produce his or her experience. The human being does not have to wait for power to fail under its own limitations, or for new narratives or social models to emerge to experience its freedom. The human animal, which is not anything determinate, not a particular kind of thing, nevertheless resists being fixed as something that it is not, and thereby 'drives' change, because – much like Bakhtin's character who will resist to the last any attempt at his or her finalization – it is not yet finished; it is still becoming. This is what power has to negotiate, and what it strives to anticipate. In its relative simplicity, in its discursively encoded operations, power works not just on the person's 'soul', or sense of self, but on and through the person as a body, with its wildly diverse flows of impulses and forces. It has to deal with something that will, on the one hand, be obedient in its search for meaning and social existence, but which, on the other hand, will at some point and in some way resist and counteract its reduction into what it ultimately cannot be: a once-and-for-all, particular, determinate thing. From the perspective of power, we are subjection-seeking beings who are simultaneously stubborn, recalcitrant, and resistant. Power must be subtle, persuasive, seductive, generous, and even underhanded, if it is to have any success in turning this awkward, overflowing, resisting being into its subject. It should also be productive rather than repressive, because the latter is more obvious, more visible, and hence more likely to evoke complaint and defiance (c.f., Foucault, 1980d). For instance, it does not tell Petra, the woman invested in romance, that she should serve the man she loves; it tells her instead about the allure of femininity. Power treads carefully, strategically, and lures us with promises rather than threats. It must operate on the basis that resistance comes first.

The idea of an embodied multiplicity of overflowing forces offers interesting possibilities in relation to the Foucauldian problem of accounting for the historical rule of social flux or change rather than social stasis. Consider the following questions:

- What mobilizes Foucault's and White's picture of an always dynamic social universe in which power is never successfully installed, but is eternally vulnerable to being destabilized? On what basis can we *know* with certainty that the social world – and the world of our clients – has not and will not become hegemonically fixed, locked in place, ordered strictly once and for all, in terms of some closed system of power?
- How do we account for the fact that, in Foucault's and White's worlds, resistance is engaged in an eternal dance with power, thereby insuring that change and flux, rather than stasis or ossification, is the empirical reality of the social world? Why does power never finally win?
- Why, in the life of the person, does power seem to need to labour, repeatedly, and in increasingly complex ways, to retain the person as a subject of its discourse? Why does it not merely mark the person with one devastating inscription, and allow this mark, in the manner of a wind-up toy, to unfold over time? Why can it not trust the person to perform his or her subjection in perpetuity?
- On what grounds do we, narrative therapists, feel assured of the universal availability of alternative discourses to those that are taken for granted; of the universal presence of implicit and de-centred experiences that do not conform to the explicit, highly visible, and centring

dominant stories; of the universal accessibility of new, creative, unexplored forms of practice? How can we be so sure that there will always be unique outcomes, that there will always be resistances, as White and Epston (1990), Wade (1997), and others assure us?

The reading I have proposed of Foucault's embodied figure and Nietzsche's overflowing bodily being allows us to bring back the individual in answering such questions. It posits change as something that we do. 'One's way of no longer remaining the same', says Foucault, 'is, by definition, the most singular part of who I am' (Foucault, 2000c, p. 444); and elsewhere, 'Do not ask who I am and do not ask me to remain the same' (Foucault, 1972, p. 17). We are impelled to change, to not stay in one place for all time, and to not be one thing forever. We are, after all, a kind of chaos, which grants us an *essential* capacity to resist.

Personally, I have found this idea of an embodied, negative form of resistance to be therapeutically useful in numerous ways, some of which I will spell out in the next chapter. It is not only that it has influenced what I say or what questions I ask in my work, but more significantly, it has allowed me to shift the emphasis of my faith in the persons who consult me: from trusting that they will always have access to lived experiences and stories to support the refusal of a particular imposed way of being, to trusting that, regardless of their access to such alternative experiences, they always have the capacity to exceed the stories imposed on them, and hence to refuse their constitution. As a therapist, I must be alert to this overflow, which corresponds to what narrative practitioners often refer to as 'unique outcomes'. Thus, if not even a fragment of experience can be found to support a new story (a rare situation, perhaps), we can know with certainty that the person is able to move away from what he or she has been made into.

I want to close this section by returning to the problem of essentialism referred to above: does my talk of actual bodies with their energies and forces take us into an essentialist position? If the post-structural rejection of essentialism involves a kind of law which says something like, 'we may not make any definitive statement about the nature of the person', what are the consequences of my argument that there is indeed *something* that lives beneath, beyond, or outside of the story? Madigan (2010), for instance, suggests there can be no such thing.

It may well be argued that the positing of a multiple, resisting body is itself an essentialist proposition – it is a kind of 'naming' after all, which says the body is 'like this' and 'not like that'. But is the claim that the body 'is multiple' the same as saying that it is definitively 'like this, and not like that'? In my view, multiplicity means that it is not 'like anything' in particular, but also that it can become 'like anything'. We should heed Wittgenstein's warning about how language can sometimes play tricks on us. So, rather than simply categorizing this argument as essentialist or non-essentialist on the face of it, let us instead engage with some of the reasons why narrative practitioners consider essentialism problematic in the first place (as discussed in Chapter 1). First, as White (1993) has indicated, essentialism threatens to introduce a 'single-voiced' account of personhood, in which the person is seen to be defined by a particular, singular, and enclosed identity (p. 135). Second, and as a consequence, essentialism tends to invisibilize alternative ways of being. And third, the view of the human being as grounded in some stable, internal essence fosters the construction of social norms and systems of control in accordance with the proposed nature of that essence. Let us briefly deal with each in turn.

First, the embodied being, by virtue of its complex and often chaotic multiplicity, is not reducible to single-voicedness, except, perhaps, by a tremendously orchestrated and aligned social system of power. But even then, as I have tried to argue, the body disrupts the hold of such impositions. Single-voicedness is simply written out as a possibility from the very beginning. To the extent that anything resembling it is found in the social world, it would be deemed a function of the reductive and simplifying dynamics of discourse and power, rather than of the body itself.

Second, the positing of a living multiplicity means that there can be no question of the invisibilization of alternative ways of being a person. The argument here is that the invisibilization of different stories and identities is a function, once again, not of the living body, but of the discourses that seek to claim it. It is discourse which has an essentializing pull, not the bodies on which it acts. Indeed, the freedom to move into alternative spaces and ways of being is already key to this embodied, multiple being.

Third, on the question of the body's essence serving as a basis for normative judgements and systems of interpersonal control, we should first note that the body of which I speak does not have any particular essential contents to which the person can be expected to adhere, or from which he or she might be seen to deviate into something like a distortion of his or her essence. His or her corporeally based recalcitrance is not a performance in the service of some essentially or universally preferred mode of being in the world, over against the modes of being afforded by society. These subversions do not (or do not necessarily) involve a particular interest in disqualifying the *contents* associated with any particular power/knowledge complex. For example, Devri does not 'contain' some a priori, embodied distaste for the system of patriarchal narratives that rationalize her husband's attempts to control her (let us refer to this as power/knowledge complex A). Nor does she contain an a priori, embodied interest in affirming a particular alternative way of being a person (e.g., her belief in human rights – power/knowledge complex B). Rather, despite Foucault's objections to something like this idea (see Foucault, 1997a, p. 75), she simply demonstrates an interest in not being captured or constrained in a totalized manner. Adapting Foucault's terminology, we can say that the soul says too little when it tries to imprison the body in its simple words and stories, and so it can never completely fulfil its socially prescribed brief. This cannot be rectified through recourse to a smarter, more efficient set of stories, because while the body finds meaning and place in these stories (as I will discuss in the next section), it also has something that no amount of storying can contain: an inclination towards the freedom of flow and multiplicity itself. Thus, power/knowledge complex B (e.g., human rights) becomes an alternative not necessarily because it is intrinsically more moral, more truthful, has better lures and is more efficient in its recruitments, is populated with better agents or relay points, or is somehow more in keeping with some imagined essential need, drive, or self. It is 'better' – at this moment, in this context and situation – because it allows the human animal to re-experience its flow; to expand just a little into its multiplicity.

This lack of essential contents tells us that the human being's multiplicity, such as I have described it, precludes any elaboration into a system of norms, forms of government, or techniques of social control, because it offers no essential, normative foundations on which these can be built, other than the requirement that we encounter them, and occasionally overcome them.

Resistance leads back to subjection

But let us not forget the positive aspect of resistance. If negative resistance is a function of our living embodiment, and has the effect of making space for the new, then positive resistance is a function of the socialized human subject, who thereby derives the capacity to fill up, or thicken these new, alternative, or seemingly unique experiences. Negative resistance cannot operate alone. In order to avoid 'dissolution and annihilation', Heidegger interprets Nietzsche as saying, we need to find a way to establish meaning, coherence, and order in the streams of our embodied existence (Heidegger, 1987, p. 85). Discourse and its machinations of power are not the enemy, as they provide our conduct, which is always embodied, with meaning. Yes, we resist them, but at the same time discourse and power offer us what Prozorov (2007b) refers to as a 'loving embrace', in the identities and social recognizability they give us, and in the sense of belonging they afford (p. 62). In a word, we need our stories.

As we have seen, the minimal, negative form of resistance – the 'no'– threatens to take the person out of discourse. But surely, one might ask, such an escape from discourse would lead to nihilism, social disconnection, and a loss of meaning? It contains no positive contents, and does not promote any particular set of values or beliefs. So, indeed, loss of identity, of social standing, and of meaning would be likely outcomes of purely negative resistance. This is where the positive, affirmative face of resistance comes in. If it is to have some effect in the social universe, and if it is to be more than a one-way trip into nothingness, the negative resistance that our multiplicity demands must be accompanied by some form of positive storying. This storying might occur in any number of ways, including the following:

- It could involve the storying of the resistance itself, an idea that might lead the therapist to pose some question along the lines of, 'How did you manage to say no?' Ensuing explorations might allow non-compliant action to be invested with meaning. For instance, White's (2007) questions assist Judy in formulating a personal story to account for how she came to step away from the culture of self-help and its prescriptions of competence and independence. Another example of this is White's curiosity about a situation between a heterosexual couple – Bette and Keith – for whom violence and control had become a problem (see White and Epston, 1990). We are told that at one point in the session, 'Bette took a risk and expressed an opinion that she knew would be contrary to Keith's' (p. 60). Ordinarily, this might have led to Keith's silencing of her, but he 'did not react'. White immediately turns to Keith and asks: 'How did you do it? I never would have predicted this at this stage'. Keith had somehow – perhaps unwittingly – made more space for Bette than would have been predicted by the discourses that governed their relationship. This action (or inaction) could then, via its storying, come to stand as resistance against these discursive requirements. Indeed, such re-storying led to the development of new accounts about Keith

(White and Epston, 1990, p. 60). But we need not assume that Keith's or Judy's resistances already existed as pre-formed stories, waiting to be unearthed by a skilled practitioner.

- In addition, the conversation might go beyond an attempt to narrate the resistance itself, to include the construction of alternative stories, which might in turn lead to the highlighting of other ways of being that have meaning for the client. For example, in Judy's situation stories develop about her Aunt Clara and the ethic of partnership, which have the potential to take her down very different paths than the stories of dependency and incompetence she had been developing. Such conversations might involve the practices of re-authoring, re-membering, and outsider-witnessing.

- But we should also consider that negative resistance can very often lead not to positive or convincing re-storying, but to the person's recuperation into the originally constituting discourse. In this instance, as we saw in an earlier chapter in the case of Nobisa, power's recapture of the resisting subject can enable power to grow, to become more effective, and sometimes more nuanced, in its subjectifying properties. Power becomes more sophisticated, in a sense it *learns*, as it tackles, strives to tame, and reinterprets resistances. It is entirely conceivable, for example, that Judy could give up trying to meet cultural requirements of independence and competence – her initial 'no' – slump into a depression, and then failing to see another way forward become motivated once more to resume her task. Here, power develops insofar as it (e.g., in her thinking or in her social circle) allows her apparent failure to be storied in ways that support the original goal: perhaps, for instance, she was not trying hard enough; or her desire to give up might be interpreted as a temporary setback, because 'real change is hard work!' And so from this point on, in Judy's life, various resistances against discourses of independence are easily reinterpreted not as protests, but as personal failures, as fatigue, as an inertia that must be overcome through willpower. Judy is thereby reinstalled as a subject of the very discourses of competence and independence she once resisted. In the absence of positive, thick storying, negative resistances become especially vulnerable to such recapture.

So, my suggestion is that the person's escape from discourse leads to a kind of vacuum of social location and meaning, and that this impels the person to move towards discourse once more. Re-storying is necessary for the person to continue to be a participant in the social world, and to retain some kind of meaning-sense of who he or she is within that world. We must become subjects once more, even if it is to be a subject in the previously resisted stories. Blunt refusal must be converted into some kind of affirmation. 'I am not this; this is not me; I do not want this' must at some point be followed by 'I am that; that is more like me'. But the latter should not be conflated with the former.

I suggest that when Foucault refers to the social 'models' necessary for agency and resistance, and White (2004) to the 'materials lying about in society' (p. 103), social presences which the individual cannot originate himself or herself, they are referring to this latter 'yes', positive story-ing, aspect of resistance. But it often relies on some kind of 'no' – some refusal of what is – which is often an individual process, not necessarily shaped by such sociocultural dynamics.

A final note on agency

I think it has become clear, in this and previous chapters, that we cannot sustain a conceptualization of agency as the sole property of the forces of social constitution (the extreme constitutionalist position), nor as the sole property of the sovereign, self-determining individual who shapes up worlds (the extreme humanist, individualistic perspective).

Interestingly, Krause (2008) argues that agency is more of a dis-tributed than localizable phenomenon. As such, I do not deny that what we call 'personal agency' is inevitably also a social achievement. Personal agency, after all, requires more than merely the troubling of discursive capture. Positive resistance – the storying of resistance; fill-ing it with contents – requires a host of visible or invisible partners for its achievement. There must in the first place be some form of dis-course, which already implicates others insofar as discourse is a socially deployed and aligned system of meanings and practices. Also, as White and other narrative practitioners have shown us, this personal storying process is significantly supported by present and absent communities, who not only uphold the person's preferred identities, but also join in its performance. In this sense, agency is a shared, socially distributed phenomenon.

In addition, our intentions associated with resistance and agency must in some way correspond to, be capable of meeting up with, the spe-cific worlds in which we live. Devri's intention to leave her husband fits only to the extent that alternative avenues (e.g., separation or divorce) are available to be explored. But the fit of our agency with the world goes beyond the social. Malafouris (2008), for example, shows how a potter's intentions are inevitably shaped by the limits and affordances of the clay material he or she works with. There are different views on this, and I do not want to go into detail on this subject, but it is interesting to note that some would see (in this example) agency itself as distributed between the potter and his or her clay; the properties of both are required for the creation of a pot. Bennet (2005), for example, sees agency as an 'assemblage' of materially existing 'actants', which themselves extend beyond the social to include whatever materially existing objects we encounter in the world.

Surely, agency is a distributed phenomenon. However, we should not allow this to cloud our vision of the individual's inherent agentive capacities; those embodied powers that he or she brings to the table. And so my focus here has been on one identifiable piece of this distributed or collective agency. The proposals I have offered here introduce an individual who seeks out discourse as an embodied being, and is therefore vulnerable to being seduced, utilized, and taken advantage of by power, but who can never be totally taken over by it. I have taken neither the strong constitutionalist nor the sovereign individualist approach, but instead tried to argue that the individual human being has a capacity for personal agency insofar as his or her embodiment allows him or her to have effects in the world that are personally meaningful. In the next two chapters I discuss how we might take advantage of this capacity for resistance and personal agency in the therapeutic dialogue.

6
Narrative Empathy and the Resisting Figure

In the previous chapter I offered a view of the human being in terms of a living body grounded in its corporeality, which affords it an inherent capacity for resistance, and propels it inexorably forward towards new forms of subjection. I see this resisting capacity as a foundational aspect of personal agency, and this belief, I have argued, does not collapse our thinking into essentialism or naïve individualism. The embodied, resisting being also has the advantage of not having to rely on discourse for its own possibility; human resistance is not dependent on an enabling discourse or pre-existing social models. This notion has the potential to help deepen our conceptualizations of several areas of narrative practice.

In this chapter, I wish to develop some of these ideas in the service of building a post-structural-narrative account of empathic engagement. I present the argument that a narrative style of empathy – listening to and reflecting what one hears from the *constituted* subject – can usefully bring us closer to the resisting, disequilibrating aspect of the human being.

Meeting the constituted subject

How do we find the constituted subject? The person's experience of being constituted in ways that include being stuck, paralysed, or without choices, is not always coherently or consistently represented in the ebb and flow of the therapeutic conversation. As therapists, we hear people intermingling talk of their problematic experiences with a range of other ideas and expressions that do not always cohere with their accounts of their problems. Even as the person identifies with certain social constructions, his or her talk and meaning-making activity will typically reveal what discourse analysts refer to as 'variation' (Potter and Wetherell, 1987). While Potter and Wetherell have in mind the multiplicity of socially available narratives and practices, we should remember also the view of the embodied human being as already constituted by a multiple array of bodily forces, which often overflow or exceed the centring, fixing tendencies of any particular discourse. Thus, for both discursive and embodied reasons, when a person speaks to a certain theme, we can expect that a range of other themes will be hinted at, picked up, and dropped off. Some of these exceptions to the problem-saturated discourse point to unique outcomes, and to the possibility of alternative constructions. We will come to that later. But for now I wish to emphasize what has come to be the reverse of much of our narrative and discursive thought: not the unique outcomes or sparkling moments, but the thrust and themes of the very problem-saturated talk that is interrupted by these exceptions. How easy it is, when in a flowing dialogue, to lose the thread of the person's constitution itself. Part of the challenge in meeting the constituted subject is to locate this thread.

Twenty-one-year-old university student, Gareth, told me about his experience of being isolated and alienated from the small group of male friends with whom he lived. He felt ostracized and had a sense of not belonging. He went on to tell me that these young men had an aggressive and disrespectful way of talking about people and animals that he could not relate to. For example, they would make crude racist and sexist comments about certain lecturers and students, and they laughed when they hit and killed a bird with their car. Hoping he could change some of this, he summoned the courage a few times to object to the ways they characterized these persons and animals, but found that this led to him being the target of their mockery and humour. He felt even more excluded and miserable. In this situation, Gareth experiences himself in the form of outsider. This is the unwanted experience for which he sought help, and in which he is caught up.

Of course, in narrative fashion we might show some interest in his summoning of the courage to confront his friends, precisely because it seems somehow in a different realm of meaning to his sense of being isolated and ostracized, and of not belonging. As a potential unique outcome, the intentional courage Gareth displays does not stand precisely in opposition to such fears and anxieties, but represents an opening into a different way of orienting to his friends, and indeed, to himself (e.g., from valuing inclusion to valuing speaking up or moral courage). But let us for the moment leave aside the possibilities of that out-of-phase interaction, noting it as something we might come back to. For now,

I am interested to stay with Gareth in his constitution as an isolated and unhappy outsider.

The implication of Gareth's original concern of being an outsider, and feeling isolated from his friends, is that he would like to be less isolated, and perhaps a more integral member of the group. However, in discussing this, Gareth expressed various seemingly contradictory ideas. He wanted to be liked and respected by these men; but he didn't like or respect them or their behaviour. He wished they would include him more when they arranged get-togethers; and he wanted to have nothing to do with them. He wanted to be included in this group as a friend; and he wanted a totally new set of friends. This complex muddle of meanings and understandings should not be seen as error or disturbance in Gareth's thinking, or as evidence of some kind of psychological ambivalence. Rather, this is almost certainly how we ordinarily talk about and live our lives. Such narrative messiness is an inevitable effect of our inherent multiplicity as well as our existence as multi-storied or multiply constituted beings.

The narrative therapist is well versed in such discursive multiplicity, and might have no difficulty in seeing these as representing different constructions of events, each of which has the potential to lead to different ways of being and doing things. Nevertheless, it is evident that constituted forms of practice and experience do have a kind of experiential coherence and integrity. Discourse's centring effects on the person's overflowing embodiment prevents him or her from *experiencing* an ability to move freely about available positioning options. After all, power in the form of social alignment functions to produce and reproduce us as particular discursive subjects. Discourse aims not at multiplicity, diversity, and variation, but at coherence, integrity, and centredness (Laclau and Mouffe, 2001). And in the previous chapter we encountered Klossowski's (2005) view that knowledge is inherently conservative, functioning to produce order, sameness, and repetition. But, as we see with Gareth, this orderedness is not always evident in the messiness of people's narrations of their experiences. Constituted experiences might feel whole, coherent, repetitive, self-identical, and inescapable, but the words and expressions used to convey them often spill over the confines of the constituting discourse, sometimes flowing into other narratives and positions in the person's experience, and so tend to be less disciplined. Coherent personal experiences are often associated not with narrative consistency, but with narrative heterogeneity.

Durrheim (1997), for instance, has demonstrated that there is considerable variability in 'right wing', 'fascist' talk in a South African context, such that racist talk is intermingled with talk of tolerance. Similarly, other discourse analysts have shown that racist, sexist, and other forms of prejudicial talk are often obscured by denials of prejudice and sometimes even favourable expressions about the objects of their derision. Think of the 'I'm not racist, but...' position that can be so easily adopted (c.f., Chiang, 2010). Some suggest that all of this observed variation is organized at some higher, central level in the person's psyche, where a single, overarching purpose or belief can be found. For example, we might imagine that the variation in a particular person's talk conceals some 'true' racist or other prejudicial attitude which is masked for rhetorical purposes, such as to make a good impression. But we should be careful not to automatically position the speaker (e.g., of racist, sexist, or any other kind of talk) as the bearer of some stable internal attitude, some inner single-voice organizing the observed multiplicity of voices, strategically manipulating his or her talk for intentionally or even unconsciously constructed purposes. Of course, it is often the case that a speaker will fashion his or her talk to come across in favourable ways. But we should recall that the human being is always multiply constituted in two sets of ways: as an embodied individual who is already multiple and thereby inclined to overflow the discursive restraints of a particular position (e.g., as racist), and as a subject produced and shaped by competing social discourses and practices. So the person is liable to speak in variable, seemingly contradictory ways, regardless of his or her intention to highlight or conceal certain opinions or beliefs. We are never fully or finally constituted, and so, as Laclau and Mouffe (2001) argue, we should be cautious of a structuralist 'essentialism', entailing 'a search for the underlying structures constituting the inherent law of any possible variation' (p. 113) – a mythical, internal, structural law which seems to unite the diversity of our talk and action. The inevitable slipperiness and variability of talk should not be seen as a cover for some hidden psychological centre or essence.

So, as we talk, some of our homogeneous personal experiences become embedded in a heterogeneous array of stories. Hence, the problem *experience* – the strong and consistent sense of this 'thing' that is wrong in the person's life – is not supported by a single, unified problem-saturated narrative. This is evident in Gareth's talk. On the one hand, his story of wanting to be liked and respected by these men relates powerfully to his unwanted sense of being an outsider. This is why he came to therapy; he has been troubled by this sense, and is ready with a host of examples from his childhood that support a reading of himself as 'always' having been something of an outsider. This is the strong, consistent, centred theme of his concerns. But his desire to challenge his peers, or even to have nothing to do with them, seems to overflow the problem story. And whether this spilling over is due to the performing body's multiple energies and forces (as we saw in Chapter 5) and/or the multiple discourses on offer in the social domain (as we saw in Chapter 4) – and I am not sure they can be easily teased apart, empirically – it nevertheless offers opportunities for the development of a range of alternative stories.

We should not expect the person's primary concern – 'I don't belong; I wish I wasn't such an outsider'; 'I am incompetent and dependent'; 'I am a failure as a man' – to be coherently and consistently followed through in all of his or her words, expressions, and stories. However, I argue that it can be useful for therapists to track these primary concerns, in among the range of other expressions and stories, and to follow them through in terms of some of the dimensions of the constituted subject articulated above, even though this is not typically the direction taken by narrative practitioners (we tend to prefer to follow the stories of unique outcomes). I suggest that it can be helpful to assist in the development of a coherent narrative around the problem itself, starting from the problem experience, in order to give some meaning to the person's sense of himself or herself. In this way, we assist not only in the articulation of a more or less coherent narrative of the problem experience, but also of the person's precise positioning within that narrative. I have been struck on several occasions in my practice that it is often during such articulation – a thickening not only of unique outcome stories, but of stories of the person's *constitution*, of his or her problem-saturated situation – that resistance is evoked, and the problem's hold destabilized.

In order to move in this direction, we need to reflect on how, and to what, we listen.

Listening to the constituted subject

The art of listening is important for any therapeutic approach, and narrative therapy is no exception. But it is clear that the notion of empathic listening, usually associated with humanistic or person-centred therapeutic approaches, is downplayed in narrative therapy. This may be associated with White's (e.g., 1997) critique, following Foucault, of the culturally prevalent 'repressive hypothesis' (p. 221), according to which the liberation of one's 'true feelings' is seen to contribute to the attainment of fulfilment, normality, and mental health. Listening in narrative therapy is not about the therapeutic identification and release of repressed feelings, and it is certainly not geared towards the attainment of some standard of normality or the discovery of one's true self. So, what is it about?

'We try to put ourselves in the shoes of the people we work with', say Freedman and Combs (1996), 'and understand, from their perspective, in their language, what has led them to seek our assistance' (p. 44). These authors go on to say that we ask questions, and we 'genuinely listen to and value people's responses, *their* ideas, not ours' (p. 277, emphasis in original). Of course, the humanist therapist also strives to get into 'the shoes' of his or her clients, but there is a difference. While the humanist might convert the person's talk and behaviour into the emotional language of therapy (e.g., using feeling words rather than words conveying facts), Freedman and Combs emphasize the client's actual words, stories, and expressions. We listen to '*their* ideas, not ours', in a quite literal sense; their ideas, in their words, in their storylines, in the terms of their knowledges; not ours. At this level, we try not to translate, and we do not assume that feelings or emotions are the universal language of human experience. This focus on the person's words comes through in our note taking too: it is recommended, for instance, that one way of practising our listening is by writing down clients' words as our therapeutic notes (Winslade and Hedtke, 2008, p. 7). We do not write down our own expert diagnoses or formulations, the feelings we hear expressed, the unconscious desires that lurk beneath the surface, or the cognitive distortions implicit in talk. Instead, we write using the very language of the client, and this becomes our therapeutic material. Indeed, my own therapeutic notes are mostly comprised of verbatim sentences and words uttered by clients (interspersed with some of my own thoughts for questions). We listen, quite literally, to our clients' stories, and their own ways – metaphors, expressions, images, meaningful words – of telling these stories.

But there is more to it than this. Therapy involves moving beyond merely hearing and noting clients' words. Much of our listening is framed in terms of what White (2003) referred to as 'double listening' (p. 30). This is the practice of listening to at least two kinds of stories at once, and as such entails a recognition and utilization of the heterogeneity of storytelling I referred to earlier. First, we listen closely to what is explicitly being said. But second, we listen to what is implied in those explicit expressions. While the explicitly told stories are often problem-saturated, the implied stories or story fragments have the potential to produce different possibilities for action or storying. For example, a person's explicit stories about the powerlessness associated with being bullied may carry with them implicit, not yet developed, stories about his or her opposition to bullying and a valuing of fairness and respect for others. Recognition of this can allow the therapeutic dialogue to move from the person's sense of powerlessness conveyed in the explicit story, to a more agentive, albeit only implicitly expressed, interest in taking a stand against bullying. The narrative practitioner listens out for these 'absent but implicit' stories that 'lie beyond the problem story' (Carey, Walther, and Russell, 2009, p. 319), and which might lead us to unique outcomes and new possibilities for identity and action.

In light of our discussion of the embodied resisting figure in the previous chapter, I want to add to this practice of double listening a way of attending to the problem experience itself. However, in this approach the question of how we listen is more complex than simply assuming that we should listen empathically: we introduce a shape, a bias even, in our listening. The notion of discursive variation – referring to the disjunction between the person's problematic experiences, which are often experienced in more or less unified ways, on the one hand, and the complex array of stories and versions of events he or she tells, on the other – is useful, if we remember that we have to work to find the coherence of the former (experience) in the multiplicity of the latter (the telling).

In my experience, clients often find it useful to develop a meaningful story of the problem itself; a set of experiences which while experientially thick, are not always very well storied. I think there are two main reasons why it might be beneficial to work at lending the messy story – even a problem-saturated story – a degree of coherence and narrative sharpness. First, it can aid in making the invisible visible. As already noted in some detail in Chapter 2, the power tactics surrounding the constituted subject are typically not immediately visible. But their operations can be made visible when we carefully develop the problem-saturated story in its own terms; in its own discourse. What might emerge, then, if we thicken the problem story, not to search for the absent but implicit, but for the manner of the person's recruitment, the way in which he or she recirculates the problem discourse in story and in action, the ways in which he or she is installed within a community of subjection, and the ways in which he or she is positioned in the story?

The second advantage I see in the articulation of a person's constitution is that it can take us towards the experiential centre of his or her problem-saturated situation: his or her subject-positioning in discourse. I suggest that in the process, we reach towards a kind of nexus, a meeting point, between the discursively constituted subject on the one hand, and the disequilibrating, disrupting, resisting being on the other. It is here that the overflowing multiplicity of which I spoke in Chapter 5 might be rendered salient. I think of this as the bringing together of identity-fixing stories and positions from the one side, and the troubling, destabilizing propensities for resistance that lurk already in the corporeally energetic and pre-discursive human figure, from the other. This is where the articulated knowledge of 'How...I become what I am' (Nietzsche, in Miller, 2000, p. 72), experienced as the heart of oneself, encounters that other 'most singular, part of who I am' (Foucault, 2000c, p. 444): one's capacity to resist or exceed what one has become.

This is what this chapter is about: attending carefully to the person's experience as a constituted subject, so that certain constitutive power relations might be exposed, and resistance evoked.

From double to single listening and back again

The possibility of staying with the constituted rather than the unique outcome story first developed in my thinking when I was working with Oscar (some of whose story I outlined in Chapter 2). When I was listening to him, I was struck by his sense of inadequacy as a man, and his increasingly rich descriptions of this. But in the spirit of double listening I noticed several other things that I, as a narrative therapist, felt I should attend to. For instance, despite feeling hopeless and lost, he had decided to come to therapy. Sometimes the very act of coming to therapy can entail a kind of resistance against accepting an unwanted sense of oneself and one's life situation. In this case, coming to therapy implied that he had not settled on his sense of hopelessness. In addition, he had met and fallen in love with another woman who was very different from his abusive ex-wife, Alice. I wondered if this step implied that he had not totally written himself off, and perhaps that he believed at some level that he was still worthy of partnership with a woman. He also at one point took several innovative steps to provide support to other men who had been in abusive relationships, which I thought had the potential to open up space for less restricted ways of thinking about what it means to be a man. All of these developments seemed somehow out of phase with, indeed they seemed to overflow Oscar's sense of being 'a failure of a man', 'incompetent', 'pathetic', and 'weak'.

But when I tried to speak to him about these things, something went wrong. My questions seemed to pull Oscar away from his current experience of distress, hopelessness, and weakness. Instead of facilitating hope, my questions left us with a sense of disconnection. I felt I had lost him, and feared that he thought I wasn't really listening. My double listening had become too one-sided, the conversation became sluggish, and Oscar seemed unable to seriously engage with openings into other narrative possibilities.

I do not deny that another practitioner might have been more prudent or more skilled in drawing out absent but implicit meanings. In any event, I utilized my avenues of peer supervision, and heard others' thoughts about my practices. But what niggled at me was how frequent an occurrence this was with a range of clients, at least in my own work. Sometimes my curiosity about these barely visible openings into new life territories led to the person's confusion at my questions, and sometimes to my own sense that I was losing touch with his or her concerns. For many years I wondered if I was moving too soon, running ahead of the person instead of staying with him or her. I wondered if my grammar was not quite right when I asked questions: externalization practices, for example, often involve a disciplined grammatical re-organization of ordinary speech, such that 'I am miserable' might become 'Misery has me in its grip'. But I found such wordings awkward and uncomfortable, and some of my clients responded with confusion and quizzical expressions. I wondered if I had fundamentally misunderstood something, and began to feel I was simply not cut out to be a narrative therapist.

It was in reflecting on this case that I decided I could not simply accept, after more than a decade (at that time) of thinking myself a narratively oriented practitioner, that the problem was my failure to do narrative therapy 'properly'. If it was the case that it was something about me that was 'wrong', then I had just about had enough of trying to be a narrative therapist. And yet I was committed to the worldview associated with this approach, particularly its emphasis on post-structural thought and the challenge of working with people to question the forms they had been assigned by societal discourse and power operations. I was energized by implications of the notion that power tends to disqualify or downgrade local knowledges. I was drawn to the idea that a sound practice would not entail the handing down of expert wisdoms from my elevated therapist position, but the privileging of these disqualified, local, and personal ways of knowing and being. Narrative therapy was clearly, I thought, a place in which I could find my therapeutic or professional home. But, strangely, I did not feel at home with many of its practices. And so I began to wonder if there could be different ways to be a narrative practitioner.

So, my conversations with Oscar had gone wrong and left us somewhat disengaged from each other. I decided to set double listening aside for a while, and to focus instead on his current experience in a more singular, one-dimensional way; to defer attention to the more hopeful implications of what he was saying and doing. But curiously, my listening seemed to have its own emphasis: I found that I was not listening in the way one normally associates with active or empathic listening (e.g., in some of the humanistic literature). I was not listening for emotion talk, I was not trying to reflect what it was like for him, and I was not trying to identify the felt sense of his current experience. It seemed that my theoretical orientation to the notions of discourse, power, narrative, the Foucauldian subject, and so on, nudged my listening in a particular direction. In particular, I found myself attending to the subject positions Oscar seemed to occupy in the stories he was telling me. When I reflected on our meetings, it occurred to me that I had been orienting less to the question 'what is this like for you?', and more to the question *'who are you in this story?'* This does not mean I consider the first question unimportant – far from it. Any therapeutic work relies on an attempt to understand what it is like for the person(s) sitting in front of us. But in many ways Oscar already knew the answer to that question: he was already telling me what his experiences were like for him. They were hard, shameful, humiliating, and disappointing. The second question, on the other hand, posed more of a challenge: 'Who are you in this story?' I was moving from listening out for experience, to listening our for implicit identity positions.

My orientation to this question ended up being very productive. Initially, I posed the question not because I thought it would be especially helpful. I had already found us to be stuck and disconnected when I had oriented to the absent but implicit aspects of his story, so I knew I had to do something else. I focused on this particular question because, first, I hoped to 'find' him once again, to reconnect, and thereby to allow our work to proceed; and second, as a post-structural, narrative, discursive thinker, I was curious about how he was positioned in the stories he was telling. I wondered if such a focus might provide a platform, or what White (2007) calls a 'reflecting surface' (p. 46), for us to understand a number of other things, such as those social forces and knowledges that prescribed this position, the kinds of behaviours it promoted, the communities which held him to this version of self, the normative notions and practices associated with it, and the ways of knowing and doing that had been disqualified (as discussed in chapters 2 and 3). In other words, I felt it might be useful to try and clarify where he lay in the power/knowledge field in which he had become trapped. So, I tried to grasp the key plot lines, the main characters, the power dynamics, and his own place in the stories he was telling me. I was pleased to experience a renewed sense of connection when I focused on trying to understand who he was in the stories he was telling me.

So there emerged a simple idea: if I want to 'meet' the constituted figure, I could begin listening out for him or her in the narrative itself. Narrative researcher Michael Bamberg (e.g., 2004) tells us that when people tell stories they organize and build whole worlds of events, experiences, moralities, objects, and subjects, including characterizations and positioning of others, all of which implicate self-construction. In other words, the person's subject positions are always somewhere in their stories, either implicitly or explicitly. Given this, let us imagine: Oscar is telling me a story that matters a great deal to him. In the telling, I hear about his 'abusive' ex-wife, his 'ashamed and disappointed' father, and his own sense of shame and humiliation; I hear about 'other men' who would never have allowed themselves to be abused, and about 'weak' men like himself who could never stand up to their women partners; I also hear about an intimidating salesman, who made Oscar feel small. The implication of Bamberg's point is that Oscar tells these stories as narrator/author, but also as a character within them. Hence the significance of the question: 'Who is Oscar in the stories he is telling?' Partly, I want to find that seemingly centred place so that I can meet him at the apparent core of his self-experience, and so that he feels met and heard.

But there is another effect of such meeting, which I only recognized much later: in arriving at that phenomenological centre – as I described it in Chapter 3 – the person's inherent multiplicity seems to become more salient, more laden with significance, which in turn enables the destabilization of power and its centripetal, experience-consuming effects.

Let us take some examples from my work with Oscar to illustrate. Oscar felt vulnerable, and became infuriated with his own inability to 'fight back' in the face of hostility. He told me about a salesman who had intimidated him. Oscar had tried to return to the store a CD player that was not working. The salesman suggested in rather forceful manner that Oscar had damaged the CD player and so he would not be refunded. Oscar felt embarrassed, and did not know how to handle this unexpected aggression. This was meant to be a straightforward exchange. Now, there are many aspects of this story I could 'hear' and focus on. I could have emotionally reflected: 'you felt intimidated by his aggression?'; or, maybe even closer to his experience in the moment of the telling, 'did you feel disappointed in yourself for not standing up to him?' But I wanted to get a better grasp of who he was in this story, and I needed to find a point of entry. I thought an external vantage point might be a useful route into this conversation, reasoning that such a per-spectival shift might artificially lift him out of the heterogeneity of his own storytelling, and allow him to imaginatively adopt the apparently singular viewpoint of the observing other (the salesman). I thought this move from a self-as-experienced to a self-as-observed position might provide Oscar with a useful distance from the self I was asking him to describe.

So I asked him how he thought the salesman saw him. He responded that the man didn't take him seriously at all. 'He seemed to think he could just push me aside, like a flea', Oscar said. I then tried to sum up my understanding – offering a version of 'editorial' (White, 2007, p. 46) (although White uses this not to refer to the person's subjection, but to his or her unique developments) – and to communicate some of my early glimpses into who he might be in the story. I offered the following thought:

> That's really tough. You already feel like you're not a real man, and now here is somebody (the salesman) in a way saying to you, in front of other people, saying to you 'I can <u>see</u> you're not a real man – you're like a flea – so I can probably push you around'. Is that it? That must be a terrible position to be in.

Oscar looked down, brooding over this, and said it was true. He told me that the man could probably see 'from a mile away' that he was 'a pushover'. I asked how the salesman could have known this about him: 'How could he have read the signs about who you were?' At first Oscar said he didn't know, but he guessed it might be to do with how he carries himself: 'I look down a lot and avoid eye contact.' I reflected:

> As a weak man, you are supposed to bow your head, look away, don't look him in the eye? That's how weak men, pushovers, men who can be swiped aside like fleas, that's how they carry themselves. Something like that?

Oscar kept quiet in response but nodded, which I took to be a silent acknowledgement that this was something close to his experience of himself.

My intention in asking these hard questions, and offering these observations, was simply to try and find Oscar – to find the horrid place he occupied – in the story he was telling me. His responses suggested to me that I was approaching something like his problem-saturated, experiential centre, the subject position around which these particular stories revolved. His responses – looking down at the floor, wordless nodding – reminded me of how people sometimes respond when a shameful secret they had been keeping to themselves was brought out into the open. I wasn't reflecting anything 'deeper' than the person I understood him to be in the explicit stories he was telling; and yet the act of trying to name his position in those stories somehow seemed to expose something that had not yet been clearly visible. Perhaps the audience of one (i.e., me) compounded his sense of exposure. And yet I had the sense that his responses were not merely about the public exposure of his 'failings' (i.e., to me). I had the sense that somehow he felt exposed to himself; as if what I had said was something he already knew, but only dimly. Perhaps he had not realized the *extent* of his position in the stories he was telling me. (As we shall discuss below, there are good reasons for this relative invisibility.)

I also sought to locate Oscar in his narratives when he was telling me about his difficult interaction with his father. Oscar had earlier told his father that he had been abused and beaten by his ex-wife – his first ever admission of this abuse to anyone. Initially, Oscar was pleased that he was beginning to voice what had happened to him, seeing this 'speaking up' as a first step against the abuse. But later on his father asked him some pointed and critical questions that undermined his positive sense of having spoken up (as mentioned in Chapter 2): 'how does a man *allow* that to happen?' After listening to Oscar's account of this painful confrontation, I responded:

> So as I understand it, you took a chance, you stick your neck out, you tell your dad about your pain. And it feels like you're doing something empowering, something good. But then he tells you 'No, this isn't good, you're not a real man…you're a weakling' (Oscar nods in agreement). Is it something like this: just when you think maybe you're not a failure as a man after all, he tells you 'No, you definitely are!' I wonder, does it seem like that's what he was saying to you?

Oscar said yes, and said it was so unfair of his father to say that. I reflected that it must have been very painful.

Looking at both instances, I was able to further reflect my understanding of who he was in this story; of the position to which he was being held by others, and which he found familiar but distressing:

> It seems to me from both of those situations, you sometimes get a distance from that sense of yourself as a failure of a man, but then sometimes other people – like the salesman and your father – can pull you right back into that position. And it seems like those invitations are somehow irresistible. It's like that's where you belong, that's who you are: a publicly visible, obvious, terrible failure of a man. That's what I understand from this, am I close to what is happening for you?

'That's who you are...' Oscar had a powerful response to this: 'That's exactly it! Yes it's so strong, I almost can't resist it, I can't stop it!' The narrative practitioner will no doubt recognize in this response the importance of the small spaces for alternative storying that Oscar was opening up: for instance, it was now merely 'almost' – not entirely – irresistible; and he maintained that his father's diminishing response was unfair. But such unique outcomes are not our concern here. Rather, I want to emphasize that these reflections seemed to resonate with his sense of who he was in the story.

We might think of Oscar's enthusiastic response in terms of what White (2007) has called 'katharsis', which he spells with a 'k' in order to distinguish it from cathartic notions of energy release or the expression of suppressed emotion (p. 194). According to White, katharsis refers to an experience that moves the person, 'not just in terms of having an emotional experience, but in terms of being transported to another place' (p. 195). Clearly, White does not have in mind the point I am making here. Nevertheless, I feel we can still think of Oscar's hearing of my reflections in terms of his being 'transported to another place'. This though, in my interaction with Oscar, is not a place of the new perspectives and meanings White is intending. Rather, he is transported to the very place which he already occupies, but which has been rendered fuzzy and indistinct by the significant noise of the heterogeneous range of stories and discourses, including those of masculinity, through which he spoke of his life.

My recognition of his narrative position is not to be confused with my telling him what he is thinking or feeling; my statement – using some of his words, his expressions, but also his sense of things – is always a question that assists us both to begin to recognize what was up until that point not clearly seen. I found that it was useful, in other words, to pay attention to the constituted shape assigned to Oscar, because at least initially, his problem-saturated, even self-loathing experience has a centred quality to it. It is a narrative or discursive centre, with a centring motion or effect (c.f., Laclau and Mouffe, 2001); pulling Oscar's experiences of life into orbit around it. In a sense, it is this active, interpellating, *phenomenological centre* that I was looking for.

I want to remind the reader that the person should not be seen as a centred being in any ontological sense (as noted in previous chapters). Indeed, in narrative practice we are committed to the idea that persons are always multi-storied. We have a decentred rather than centred understanding of identity. We know that a range of subject positions, stories, and practices are always available to us, meaning that any one identity position – any particular sense of oneself – is never truly centred as the cause or driver of one's conduct. There are always others jostling for representation, and so any form of identity can in principle be destabilized. And, as discussed in the previous chapter, the embodied human being, by virtue of his or her inherent multiplicity, is in any case always already a decentred being, who refuses to be tethered to one centred position, and retains an innate ability to move through and beyond discursively imposed identity forms. However, the ontological reality of selfhood – understood here in terms of both its inherent multiplicity and its simultaneous subjection to multiple possible discursive formations – should not be confused with the person's experience of himself or herself. Very often the person experiences himself or herself in an essential, monolithic, unidimensional, singular, and often unwanted way, even to the extent that escape from this position seems impossible. The person can, in other words, have a centred *experience* of himself or herself – 'I am a loser', 'my life is hopeless', 'I am a schizophrenic', 'I'm ugly, that's just who I am'. These descriptions can feel like they refer to something existing at the very core of the person's being. Our theoretical knowledge that these descriptions are partial, thin, not fully centred, should not prevent us from recognizing that they can be *experienced* nevertheless as thick, comprehensive, central aspects of the self. When Oscar says, 'Yes, that's exactly it', he is referring to the truth, the centredness, of a particular sense of who he is. He might as well have said 'spot on, you hit the mark dead centre'. We know, theoretically, that he is decentred, but this does not lead him to say, 'Well, not quite, but close enough'. Instead, he says, 'Exactly'.

This, after all, is what successful discourses do: they dominate the social field of possible ways of thinking and being, and they seek to impose particular versions of selfhood, by constructing a centre around which persons are expected to orbit (Laclau and Mouffe, 1985). A supremely successful discourse invisibilizes or sidelines other possibilities, reducing the rich multiplicity of embodied human experience towards a kind of singularity. This can leave the person with a thickly held, deeply felt sense about who he or she is, in the terms and parameters of that discourse. And it is this (discursively constructed) central, centralized, dominant, experience of self that I found myself trying to find in order to meet Oscar as a constituted figure; to meet the person he was in those moments.

Before resuming my account of my work with Oscar, I want to briefly reflect on the curious fact that despite the powerful personal resonance of these central self-experiences – the subject positions we found at the heart of his narratives – they seemed to emerge as if they had been hidden from view.

The invisibility of subject positions

We might think that our positions in discourse are easily identified and spoken about, and sometimes this is certainly true. However, sometimes the positions that anchor us in particular narratives – positions which form a kind of central lynchpin or pivot around which narratives gain, for each of us, their personal meaning – are diffused, only vaguely perceived, and imprecisely articulated. Indeed, there is something very interesting about the way in which my positional reflections resonated with Oscar's experience of himself. Oscar recognized himself in these words; and yet at the same time they seemed to surprise him. What interests me about this – and one often comes across this in a variety of empathic practices, regardless of therapeutic approach – is that his energized response does not suggest that he was fully aware of his position all along, but just the opposite. Somehow this seemed to be a crucial piece of the story that he had not yet been able to put his finger on. A piece of the story only dimly perceived, but whose sudden articulation elicits an energetic 'Aha! That's me!' kind of response. My question is: why does it seem to come as a surprise?

If we think of this in terms of narrative heterogeneity in the context of experiential homogeneity, as discussed above, we might make sense of this as follows. Oscar, like all of us, is an embodied multiplicity who is simultaneously positioned in multiple social discourses. Thus, his talk inevitably displays variation, and does not, for instance, consistently follow the themes of masculinity or masculine failure. During the course of our many sessions, he presented himself in innumerable ways: as a loving son, a computer whizz, a protector of his sick sister, a defender of righteousness, a tough negotiator, a disinterested observer of a car accident, a good neighbour, and so on. He is many things, and occupies many positions, as is to be expected. But his *problem experience* is not as diverse as his multiple stories and positions suggest. He can briefly adopt some of these other positions, but they seem weak and inconsequential in the face of the larger problem. Indeed, in much narrative practice we have to work to render this multiplicity visible and usable, precisely because the person's problem-saturated experience blocks meaningful access to them. And so, in the context of this multitude of embodied identity practices and associated discourses, his more *singular* problem-saturated *experience* is not easily narrated. It exists in the context of the considerable noise of a range of other stories and self-understandings, many of which seem incidental to his almost monolithic experience of misery, anxiety, panic, and hopelessness; this 'thing' he wants help with.

So, in relation to the question of how personal positions are rendered invisible, and evoke surprise when articulated, my first hypothesis concerns the noise of multiple stories. The multiplicity of the person's narratives and positions effectively obscures from view the single position in which he or she is anchored by those stories which author his or her problem-saturated *experience*. And so the identification of this position in my meetings with Oscar comes as something of a surprise. We might think of this in terms of what Stern (1997) calls 'unformulated experience' (p. 33). But for our purposes we should not understand the idea of 'unformulated' as equivalent to 'unconscious', in Stern's psychoanalytic sense. Rather, Oscar's positioning is implied in, it is a narrative consequence, even a product of, the problem-saturated stories he tells. Some of the person's stories carry implications for who he or she must be in order for these stories to be true. The person does not necessarily expressly articulate this position, and so it is in this sense unformulated. Their explicit formulation might often invite resistance, especially on the part of persons who are positioned in culturally devalued ways. But these stories, nevertheless, rely on this position as a kind of invisible fulcrum for their intelligibility and performance. The position is one of the story's invisible givens. It is, in a sense, unconscious, but, to borrow again from Foucault (1998a), not 'the "unconscious" ... of the speaking subject, but of the thing said' (p. 309).

The second and related reason for the only implicit nature of these positions is that our stories are rarely about our 'selves'. The stories people tell, and the experiences they have of life, are very often not explicitly *about* themselves, but about circumstances, situations, other characters, actions, and events: bullies, lost love, injustice, or the witnessing of a horrific accident. Guignon (1993), taking a Heideggerian perspective, says that we are generally outside of our 'selves' (p. 223), meaning that the person – as actor, social participant, and storyteller – often does not formulate a meaningful or coherent sense of his or her own *place* in the stories and situations of his or her life. In the hustle and bustle of our lives, that personal position is not as salient as we might suppose. On this account, the articulation of a person's position in the stories he or she tells, which brings about a coherence or alignment between story and 'self', can seem, simultaneously, both familiar and strange.

And there is a third reason: narrative self-visibility can be costly. Foucault (1998b) asks an interesting question about the positioning effects of discourse: 'At what price can subjects speak the truth about themselves?' (p. 444). O'Leary (2002) offers part of an answer: 'at the price of being (self-)constituted as a particular kind of subject, at the price of being tied (by oneself and others) to a particular identity' (p. 113). So, what is the price Oscar must pay in speaking the truth about who he is (i.e., the truth according to the terms of these stories)? It seems to me that for him to do so – to name himself as, in the end, a failure, a shameful excuse of a man – might prove very costly indeed, both personally and socially, as O'Leary suggests. While he is perpetually aware, in a lived and experiential way, of the sense of masculinity and his numerous failures to meet up to its standards, his sense of what this says about him – about his identity or 'self' – remains thinly narrated, a fuzzy possibility in his self-awareness. This self-awareness tends to be more a background question ('could I really be that?') than a foregrounded conclusion ('I am that'). We have already seen that it can be easily clouded by multiple positioning in the complex task of living life, and by his orientation to the world around him rather than to his 'self'. But there is also a level of risk involved in the articulation of his position relative to the problem discourse, which might contribute to his reluctance to become aware of the deadening identity conclusion in a narratively precise way.

Let us speculate: what would happen were Oscar to *know*, in a precisely, explicitly articulated way, that this is the essential truth about his self; that it is *true* that he is a hopeless, embarrassment of a man? If this is the truth (and I mean here narrative rather than ontological truth), if this is who he must be for the problem-saturated stories of his life to be true, then he might come to the following conclusions: that the multiple alternative positions he otherwise adopts, as well as many of his multiple and variable bodily experiences and social performances, are merely self-assuring lies, fictions concealing the devastating truth of who he 'really is'; and that, therefore, his situation is more hopeless than he had thought, all escape routes (e.g., into other ways of being and experiencing) having now been disqualified as untrue, as defensive, as myths. So in terms of Foucault's question about the price he would have to pay for speaking this (narrative) truth about himself, Oscar is better off referring to it and thinking it only in vague, fuzzy ways, and only in the fleeting moments of his most intense self-loathing. He is better off giving himself at least some space to breathe into his multiplicity, to occasionally move on to experiencing and presenting himself as a loving son, a caring brother, and so on. After all, he seldom presents himself as the trembling, vulnerable, weak, shameful thing his thematic story suggests, despite his resonance with the description I offered. Recall that when he presented at the hospital after being assaulted by his ex-wife, he made up a story to the nurses and doctors precisely to conceal this 'truth' about himself, so that he could, in his words, 'look them in the eye'. So while on the one hand there is a narrative 'truth', an implication of the words and stories he is telling, and it resonates powerfully with him when it is uttered, it is, on the other hand, not one he can tell about himself, either to others or to himself, without the significant cost of becoming this one, singular, subjectified thing, which in his case is something like a jellified, useless, undesirable, and unworthy human being.

All of this brings us back to the important question: under these circumstances, why should we strive to name this otherwise dimly perceived position, in as precise a way as possible?

Naming the experiential centre: A route to resistance

We can think of the empathic naming of an experiential centre as the simultaneous articulation of a narrative constraint, in the context of an embodied individual who is always inherently multiple. Oscar, positioned as something like a 'weak, failure of a man', is more intensely constrained within that particular narrative by virtue of its very articulation. However, we have seen that the human being has the capacity to throw off or exceed the narrative constraints imposed upon him or her, even without necessarily having some alternative preference in mind. This view is supported by Bakhtin's (1984) depiction of the person as always having an 'internally unfinalizable something' (p. 58); an 'inner unfinalizability', which entails a

> capacity to outgrow, as it were, from within and to render untrue any...finalizing definition of them. As long as the person is alive he lives by the fact that he is not yet finalized, that he has not yet uttered his final word. (p. 59)

In terms of our own discourse, the therapeutic naming of the person's problem-saturated identity position seems to run counter to what Bakhtin understands to be a requirement for being alive. In fact, to use Bakhtin's words, it seems to be a way of 'degrading and deadening' the human being (p. 59). Indeed, many of Oscar's responses to my questions suggest a kind of 'deadening': he would look down at the floor, sigh, and nod without words.

Bakhtin's thesis, consistent with what I argued in the previous chapter, is that people resist such deadening. We struggle against being captured or limited in one position. Our multiplicity insures that we are always, as Bakhtin puts it, 'poised *on the threshold*' (1984, p. 63; italics in original) between one position and another, between one way of knowing oneself and another. This is all very well, but as noted above, and as we know from our work and life experience in general, this threshold is not always visible or easily accessible. Part of our function as narrative practitioners, I believe, is to promote such visibility and accessibility, and to facilitate movement towards and through that threshold, in the direction of new possibilities. And so it is relevant to note the implication of the arguments made thus far, that individuals are already threshold-dwellers, evidencing a Nietzschean 'principle of disequilibrium' relative to power, by which they bristle against, unsettle, and exceed social prescriptions and controls (Klossowski, 2005, p. 79). The view here is that people 'acutely sense their own inner unfinalizability', and when faced with restrictive forms of constitution are inclined to engage in what Bakhtin describes as 'furious battles with such descriptions of their personality in the mouths of other people' (i.e., in discourse) (1984, p. 59).

This has important implications for how we think about the therapeutic practice of empathy. It is difficult to engage in resisting activity if we are not clear on what is being resisted. There is no need to resist what Bakhtin describes as the deadening and degrading proclamation – the finalizing judgement – if it is never made. And this is where I see an important role for a post-structural, narrative version of empathy, in the form of collaborative empathic positioning. If empathic reflections and questions can assist persons in articulating certain key features of their constitution as subjects, then it is likely that such reflections and questions can help provide a narratively clear point from which resistance can be launched. We can think of this narrative point as possessing a clarity which not only makes exceptions, differences, and unique outcomes more visible, but also has the capacity to confront the person with a finalized, and hence resistance-promoting, description of himself or herself.

So with this in mind, let us return to my work with Oscar. I noted above my interest in the fact that his response to my final editorial of that session – in which I reflected on his position as a failure, and others' recognition of this – was, quite unlike his previous responses, animated and energized. His eyes lit up, his eyebrows lifted, he sat upright in his chair, and he raised his voice: 'That's exactly it!' he exclaimed. What did he have to be so energized about, given that our talk was drifting towards his finalization? Was this not a deadening reflection? Were we not making visible precisely the invisible position whose naming comes at significant cost? Why did Oscar become excited and energized, rather than descend into utter hopelessness? Why did he not succumb to the feeling that all of the things that had given him hope – his alternative ways of being a person – were revealed as lies now that the 'truth' had been named?

What looked like an answer to this question appeared early on in our following session, in which Oscar began, uncharacteristically in terms of our relationship, to question my authority in the therapeutic interaction. In an earlier session I had suggested he consider some couples' work given some of the difficulties he was having in his current relationship. Now, Oscar, appearing nervous and fidgety, told me he had been thinking about that idea, and decided I had made an 'inappropriate' suggestion, as this therapy was for him. It seemed to me he had moved from being a 'failed man' in the last few minutes of one meeting with me, to one who challenges the 'expert' advice of his therapist, in the first few minutes of the next. In the moment of his allegation of my inappropriate conduct, I experienced a stark shift in my own positioning in the interaction, the significance of which I did not appreciate at the time. At the end of the previous session, I had experienced myself as a concerned and interested listener, working respectfully to appreciate Oscar's position in his life. I was something like an appreciative partner, reaching to understand and hear him. Now, I experienced myself as someone who had specifically *failed* to appreciate, to understand,

and to hear Oscar's situation. Significantly, this was a shift (in my own positioning) initiated by Oscar's words and actions. In other words, following once more Bamberg's (2004) idea of the implicit positioning of self and other in narration, we can see this shift in my own positioning as associated with a shift in Oscar's self-positioning. Clearly, in these first few moments of our next session, Oscar was not speaking from the place of the failed man, and I had to be repositioned as a consequence. So he positioned me away from my preferred appreciative listening place, which complemented his self-understanding in the earlier session, towards the position of a failed listener, which did not. It was this shift, and my immediate response to it (I got a fright and felt uncomfortable about being reprimanded), that alerted me to the fact that something different was happening (see Guilfoyle, 2009).

When I reflected on this shift later on, I wondered if his explicit, and relatively precise positioning as a weak man in relation to certain more intimidating and judgemental others (in our previous session), had served as a platform for a different style of social engagement; such as the one we engaged in in our next meeting. Certainly, his challenging actions were lent considerable salience to both of us by virtue of the fact that we had just articulated his status as 'a terrible failure of a man'. I wondered if this stark characterization had brought him, to borrow from Bakhtin, not only to the narrative centre but also to its *threshold*; effectively situating him between one kind of position and another, which was yet to be defined. It seemed he had moved to his discursively constituted centre – a weak, failure of a man – and almost immediately overflowed it, revealing his inherent resisting capacities. It is, I suggest, the narrative clarity of this problem-saturated centre that makes it simultaneously so capturing and so vulnerable to the person's overflowing multiplicity. The clarity, structure, and tangibility of this centred position enables it to be experientially *occupied and embodied*, which in turn allows the limits of its containing function to be exposed by the individual's excess. It seemed that Oscar could only experience his exceeding of the problem-saturated description, and recognize its limitations, when he was fully interpellated into it.

Of course, one might argue that Oscar's challenging of me, calling my suggestion 'inappropriate', was merely a face-saving response to the negative position we had identified in the previous session: a simple denial of his masculine failure, and a reactive proof of his masculinity. I have two responses to this. First, the point I am making does not (yet) concern where he 'goes' with this resistance (e.g., back to masculinity, or elsewhere). I am emphasizing only *that* he resists the finalizing conclusion.

And second, this resistance should be recognized as an opportunity for re-storying, and so a renewed sense of masculinity is just one of many possible narrative trajectories. This is where the therapeutic dialogue becomes extremely important. In this regard, it is worth noting that Oscar's reference to my 'inappropriate' conduct led to a useful conversation about ways of knowing himself that had been subordinated up to that point, silenced by the hegemony of his overwhelming sense of masculine failure. A re-authoring conversation flowed out of his resistance, allowing it to gain some positive storying in the context of a range of other life experiences. In particular, we explored the ideas of masculinity that his father, his ex-wife, and many other people in that cultural setting performed. Together, we wondered whether these ways of knowing and being were fitting for what was important and valuable in his own life. One interesting thing to come from these discussions was his recognition that masculinity was 'not a big thing' for his new partner. I wondered aloud what she might say about the conversation we were having, and about his challenging of me. He decided to speak with her in between sessions about some of these issues, and reported back that she described him very appreciatively as a 'gentle, quiet soul who comes through when it counts': no mention of 'masculinity'. His opposition to my suggestion of couples' counselling would come to stand not as a proof of his masculinity in reaction to the emasculated position we had named in the previous session, but as an example of his 'coming through' for himself 'when it counts'.

As I see it, negative embodied resistances can only give us therapeutic opportunities, not the stories required for their development into something new.

Linking with re-authoring and other narrative practices

I am not recommending such finalizing empathic engagement as a substitute for other narrative practices such as unique outcome conversations, externalizing, re-authoring, or remembering. Instead, I mention this practice as something I have found useful, and which seems to cohere with the theoretical points already made. Also, speaking as a practitioner, this single listening strategy – deferring double listening, and the emphasis on unique outcomes to a later point in the process – sits more easily with the flow of my style of interacting with persons. And yet it is still a post-structural *narrative* orientation, informed, as has been extensively discussed, by Foucauldian notions of power, discourse, subjectivity, and identity. I do not consider this a more accurate reading of these notions, but as another way of making use of them. In using this practice, I have also found it very useful to conduct re-authoring conversations with people, and to work with the unique outcomes that emerge around and unsettle – or rather overflow – their centred positioning.

The integration of such listening with other narrative practices can be illustrated through my work with a 22-year-old man, named Kevin, who had been involuntarily admitted to a psychiatric hospital. He had been seen standing at the top of a tall building, and the police were called. They found him crying and threatening to jump. He was talked down, and admitted for psychiatric assessment and treatment. In hospital, he was referred to see me. In our first conversation, it emerged that one of the several issues that concerned him was the death of his friend and flatmate, Hans. Kevin told me that three years earlier, around age 19, he and Hans were out with some friends, and they both drank too much alcohol. Towards the end of the evening, Hans said they should get a lift home with somebody else, rather than drive back in Kevin's car. Kevin told me that he had ridiculed Hans for always being scared of adventure, and made sarcastic comments like, 'Yes, Hans, I'm sure your mommy would disapprove'. Eventually, Hans joined in the teasing, and laughed at himself. He said Kevin should drink some coffee before they left the party and that he'd better drive carefully. But on the way home, they had a terrible accident. Kevin does not recall exactly what happened, and thinks he may have fallen asleep at the wheel. In any event, he only remembers the car being in a ditch, with its front end smashed in. When he turned to check if Hans was alright, he saw that he was not in the car. Kevin got out and found Hans lying a few metres in front of the car, evidently having been thrown out through the windshield. Kevin says Hans was bloodied and unconscious, but breathing. Kevin called emergency services but by the time they arrived, some 15 minutes later, Hans had passed away.

It was determined that Kevin's alcohol levels were over the legal limit. This led to a court case, and Kevin was given a suspended sentence and sent for rehabilitation for excessive alcohol use. It was a few months after ending his rehabilitation programme that Kevin went to the top of a tall building, planning to end his own life.

In discussing this, I sought to clarify Kevin's position in the story he was telling and living through. The following interchange took place:

Kevin: I have to live with this, and I can't. Hans was a very trusting person, and I always led the way. He trusted me, but I led us into trouble so many times, and he always just went along with me, trusting me that everything would be ok.

Michael: This is so hard.

Kevin: If I hadn't been such a prick about it, he was right, we should have gotten someone else to take us home, but I was too busy being the big man, the arrogant shithead, stirring, laughing at him, getting him into dodgy situations.

Michael: You having to be the leader, the arrogant hot shot, the big man, all of this put Hans, trusting Hans, at risk, in terrible, grave danger.

Kevin: (Starts crying) Yes, I'm so stupid, what kind of person does that? I mean I don't deserve to live.

Michael: In a way even the court's decision of a suspended sentence...

Kevin: Well, it just lets me off the hook, doesn't it? I mean, 'manslaughter', it says you have some extenuating circumstances, lets you off the hook. I mean, yes I was relieved, but really... (pauses)

Michael: So you're relieved, but it also feels like justice wasn't done?

Kevin: Right, right. I don't want to go to prison, obviously, but...

Michael: Justice would be more like, you don't deserve to live, because you killed your best friend. He trusted you, he put his life in your hands, and you killed him. You're a killer, a murderer, and you don't deserve to live, you don't deserve to be out in the world having your own life.

Kevin: (Sobbing) Yes!

We talked some more in this manner, congruent with his sense that this is the only truthful way to understand what happened: that he is totally and utterly to blame for killing his friend. I do not contradict him on this, because at this moment I am simply trying to understand – in a constitutive sense – who he is; who he has become. So here, I suggest, we arrive in our conversation at something like the central position in which his narrative installs him. This is the principle according to which, around which, he was interpellated, and around which his talk and experience revolves. This is his position as a constituted subject – he is a murderer – and it is almost literally a 'deadening' one.

But then a few minutes later, there is a small but significant shift.

(Five minutes later)

Michael: All of this feels impossibly painful, like too much for one person to carry, and it must seem there's no way out for you, but to die.

Kevin: Yes, it's true. But now (sniffing, blows his nose) I'm just wondering, you know, a part of this is not my being an evil killer or whatever. I'm not a bad person really. It's also my being arrogant, full of myself, and, I don't know. Do you think...? No, no, no, it's far too soon, I'm just making pathetic excuses now.

Michael: Hang on Kevin, I think it could be important – you saw just there that there might be different ways of thinking about this, and I would agree with you. But is what stops you, is it that somehow it would be unfair to Hans? And too much letting you off the hook to really follow down the path of a different way of thinking about it? I heard you saying just there that you're not just an evil killer, you're not a bad person really. You were hinting that you're also something else, like an arrogant, teenage, stupid fool caught up in his own reputation, or something, I don't know what you were going to say, but I thought you were headed towards something like that.

Kevin: Yeah, yeah.

Michael: But what I understand from this is that for you right now it's just too soon to think about, to even consider other ways of thinking about this. The only thing that's okay to think now is that you're an evil killer, maybe you're just a bad person. Everything else is just excuses. Do I have it right?

Kevin: Yep, well that says it all. It says it all.

This excerpt demonstrates what I have found to be one of the significant therapeutic advantages of positional empathic engagement and understanding: it can serve to illuminate ideas, practices, and values that are not totally determined by the problem-saturated narrative. The excess becomes salient. These are fleeting impulses, ideas, practices, and values that run counter to the centring, centripetal tendencies of this narrative. In this instance, just a few minutes after reaching what seemed Kevin's central position in the story he was telling – Kevin as a bad person, a killer, a murderer – he found a glimmer of a new way of thinking about this situation: something about being 'arrogant', 'full of' himself, and maybe even '*not* a bad person'. Not all flattering thoughts, but significant in that they don't call for his death or exclusion from life in the way that his being a 'killer' does. I felt it was significant that the tag of 'killer' was now not totalizing his experience. His words tell me that it is not the only explanation for what happened, as he recognizes that there are other ways of thinking. But it is not a path he is ready to follow. It is 'too soon', and it feels like cheating, and a way of letting himself 'off the hook'. What 'says it all', for him, is not that he is a killer as such, but that this is the 'only thing that's okay to think' right now. From my perspective, that is a significant shift.

Kevin's willingness to think the most difficult thoughts had me speculating about his values in taking this stance, as often occurs when engaged in a re-authoring conversation. I wondered how we might talk about what Kevin seems to have established as a priority: accepting and facing the killer label, and not making any excuses. I became curious about his readiness to overrule the court's decision (who he felt had let him 'off the hook') in his own thinking. I wondered if his resolute facing up to (what seemed to him) the harsh truth of the situation reflected something about his personal ethics and values. Was this something he had always been able to do? But I was in two minds about expressing these questions, and in those moments I kept them to myself, because I felt sure that Kevin would see this line of conversation as a way of putting a 'positive spin' on things. And besides, in his story, the issue is not him and his values, but what he did to Hans. He would surely, in the logic of the story being told, find it distasteful to think of himself as 'bravely' (not a word I would use, but one that I feared he would hear) facing up to the truth.

So I asked him instead to tell me about Hans, and about their friendship. We sought to honour Hans in some way. This included a re-membering conversation, in which we explored Hans' impact on Kevin's life. After some talk on this, I began to wonder if there was space in Kevin's experience for images of Hans as someone who was not only the victim of a tragic accident. It struck me that this was probably a very limiting picture of Hans and his own life. So I asked Kevin if Hans' ways of being in the world, ways of being that might have come through in their relationship, had affected him during their friendship. He told me about things he loved about Hans, and occasionally stopped to cry during his telling. I asked if he thought Hans knew about the many ways in which Kevin had appreciated and loved him. Kevin said he was not sure about this. He then told me that talking about all of this made him realize that he had never had the chance to really grieve over the loss of Hans, because the tragedy had become so caught up with his own terror around the court case, his feelings of defensiveness when he saw Hans' friends and family members, his detention in a rehabilitation centre, and his own wish to die. He realized that he had not had the chance to speak to Hans 'in peace', to talk things through with him at the graveside, and to say sorry in a way that was not clouded by all these other complicating factors. Talking this way was meaningful for Kevin, who said he would like to visit the graveside and talk things over with Hans when he was discharged from hospital. We spent some time discussing what kinds of things he wanted to say.

It seemed that Kevin's guilt over Hans' death was edging towards grief. Maybe Kevin had been right that it was 'too soon' to imagine himself not a murderer, because he had not yet grieved his friend's death, and he had not yet spoken to Hans about it in a proper way. Until then, it was hard to know how he could live. But for now, he was not so much invested in ending his life as he was in speaking to Hans. His self-loathing and self-blame drifted towards apology, sadness, and grief. And his sense of himself as a murderer edged towards a recognition that he was not, in the end, a 'bad person'. He was Hans' friend, and he needed to talk to him. Until he did that, it would be hard to know what he was, or could be.

Aspects of empathic positioning practice

The practices I am proposing are not oriented to providing spaces for emotional expression or 'catharsis', in the traditional sense. Rather, I suggest that precise narrative positioning can be useful in the following respects: it promotes the person's sense that the therapist is trying to understand his or her current experience, without moving too quickly to solution-focused work; it has the potential to make unique outcomes clearer to both parties, or the range of ways in which the person's embodied conduct and speech overspills the problem narrative's positioning of him or her; and its clarity and experience-nearness can leave the person feeling contained within, and simultaneously bristling against, an unwanted, limiting, almost-but-not-quite-right, discursive position. This capture may aggravate the person into a dynamic of disequilibration or disruption; a series of moves to throw off the deadening or degrading restraints that have been imposed on him or her.

There are four further aspects of this practice that I want to highlight. First, this form of empathic engagement involves approaching and naming the subject position itself, not the feeling state or felt sense of the person's experience. We are striving to identify the subject position that declares the person's identity – in the form, 'this is who you are' – not what he or she is currently experiencing in the moment. This is the discursive point into which he or she is pressed by social forces of constitution, the perspectival vantage point from which he or she is expected to obediently speak, act, and feel. It is an 'I am' rather than an 'I feel' position.

It might be helpful to distinguish empathic positioning from the reflections of emotion, feeling states, or felt-senses one frequently hears emphasized in various therapeutic approaches. However, we should first note that the association of emotional reflection with person-centred, humanist, and existential therapies is not quite so clear-cut. Empathy was equated with the specific practice of reflecting feelings in the 1950s, but as a concept it has since expanded significantly. Carl Rogers apparently became rather irritated that such a reductionistic interpretation of his approach persisted into future decades (Worsley, 2008). In more recent years, empathy has come to be understood not merely as a specific technique or practice (e.g., reflection of feelings), but as a more general and pervasive 'phenomenological stance', incorporating an attitude of 'trying to fully enter the world of (the) client' (Haugh, 2008, p. 40). Emotional reflections have come to represent only one way of doing so.

I mention this here so that we do not misrepresent the humanistic and related traditions. My intention at this point is not to tackle those understandings of empathy, but to highlight aspects of the kind of empathic positioning I have discussed by contrasting it with other ways of thinking about empathy. Perhaps the most convenient distinction we can make here is between the phenomenonological question, 'what is it like?' on the one hand, and the empathic positioning question, 'who are you?', on the other. Consider Bohart and Greenberg's (1997) argument that there are two interrelated kinds of empathy in the therapeutic world today: one directed at the question of what 'it is like to be the client in a general sense' (e.g., through his or her personal history), and the other concerned with 'what it is like to be the client right now' (e.g., in the consulting room) (p. 425). As the reader will notice, both are concerned with the question: 'what is it like?' This focus is broad enough to permit the incorporation of reflections of feelings, but – as Rogers warns – does not narrowly limit the therapist's interventions to that domain. The therapist has scope to reflect on any number of experiential domains in order to get closer to a sense of what it is like to be that person, either right here-and-now or in a more general sense.

What I wish to emphasize here is that this phenomenological approach to empathic reflection – reaching towards a connection with what it is like to be this person – does not 'finalize' the person, in the Bakhtinian sense. Indeed, it is designed to achieve just the opposite. One of the functions of such reflections is that they tend, specifically, *not* to evoke resistance, but to foster the person's continued exploration of feelings and experiences associated with a particular theme (e.g., Zimring,

2000, p. 225). They take the person onward, if I may impose a narrative translation, further *into* the story being told. Of course, this non-finalizing trend is a helpful aspect of much empathic technique, given the understanding that the naming and exploration of a given sense of things (e.g., of guilt) is designed not to trap the person there, or to hold him or her to it, but to facilitate expression and from there, onwards towards self-awareness, growth, and self-actualization (Haugh, 2008).

However, empathic reflections orienting around the theme 'what is it like?' do not concern themselves with the theme, 'is this *who you are?*' In my view, the utility of this latter orientation lies in its inclination towards finalization, making it more likely to evoke and reveal resistance than traditional empathic communications. It is more enlivening of the principle of disequilibrium, and of the person's capacity to trouble and unfinalize such declarations and to usher in previously disqualified or alternative ways of knowing.

Consider, for instance, the therapist's empathic statement to Kevin, in the face of his guilt over the death of his friend: 'you feel very guilty'. This might be a useful emotional reflection, and it might contribute to Kevin more fully experiencing his guilt. But this kind of reflection does not refer to the person's positioning as such. It reflects what he or she is experiencing, or what it feels like to be in the situation in which he or she finds himself in that moment. Significantly, from our perspective, there is usually no need to resist the effects of such an emotional reflection statement (unless, of course, it feels untrue). First, it is experience-near and serves as a kind of affirmation of what the person is already saying. It is also evident to both parties, at least implicitly, that the truth of this feeling does not prevent the person from moving on to feeling something else at another point in time. 'Yes, I do feel guilty', Kevin might say, 'and later on today I might feel angry, or sad. And tomorrow I might forget for a few minutes and steal a few moments of laughter and happiness'. The therapist's empathic communication ('you feel very guilty') does not suggest that guilt is the only feeling, or that guilt lies at the heart of the person's identity; only that the person is, quite simply, having this experience. Therefore, a range of different experiences at other points in time – happiness, sadness, anger – cannot disqualify the guilt reflection itself. Indeed, the person's reflections on his or her guilt typically give way to a host of other experiences. In other words, the reflection allows for experiential movement and diversification, and permits an elaboration, an opening up, even an enrichment, of the personal narrative. It runs precisely counter to the finalizing, deadening, or degrading directions we have been considering.

But such freedom to move deeper into the story, to explore its range of plot lines, characters, emotional positions, and so on, is not always so readily available with a positional reflection. In the latter instance, the position, once understood, serves as a kind of final destination, its articulation rendering salient the perspectival point from which and around which the story makes sense. It can evoke only limited thickening of, or further exploration into, the current story, because, in a sense, there is nowhere else to go. It is as if we have read the final chapter of a hermeneutically sealed book (called, for example, 'You Are a Murderer'), in which the discovery of the position has left nothing to be explained, in which all the spaces for new meanings have been closed up, and in which the pieces of the narrative puzzle have been put in place. It is in this context that the person's sense of narrative capture entails a sense of finalization. This is the sense of being one definite, monolithic, isolated, trapped, self-contained thing, always and forever. The final truth has been spoken and the book can now be closed. This is why I find Foucault's question – about the dangers of telling the truth about who one is – so apt; it threatens to close life down. There are terrible prices to be paid when one speaks this truth, as Foucault rightly recognized. But I have argued that there are also significant advantages, provided that its articulation takes place in a relationship that is ultimately geared towards the unfinalization of such finalized conclusions; a relationship that recognizes this as a liminal place, and nurtures the person towards, and through, the narrative's identity conclusions.

So, if we think of this process in terms of the Nietzschean vision of a multiple body that overflows its discursive capture, and in terms of Bakhtin's thesis of the unfinalizable human being, we become alert to the likelihood that such a positional recognition will give way to its own undoing. And I wish to reiterate that this finalized identity realization is not the *therapist's* conclusion, although we assist in putting it into words. Nor is it, in the end, a conclusion about *the person* as such. Rather, it is a conclusion about the one-dimensional, caricatured figure that the story describes. As a deadening, end-of-the-line conclusion, it will not do for the living being, despite its powerful resonance and capacity to semantically organize the story's array of emotions, events, and activities. It is as if a new book, or perhaps an unexpected chapter, now calls out to be written. The living being always reaches out for new stories to be told. And so we witness the person moving to reinstall dynamism into his or her life narrative, to usher in a freedom of movement for the characters and happenings that had become constrained in the problem-saturated narrative. This is where we notice, in the consulting room, the living, dynamic human being, awakening to resist the deadening discourse.

Second, I have found it useful to build up a thick constitutive understanding in conversation with my clients, so that my positional reflections do not come out as hollow declarations. The naming of a position requires extensive rationalization and justification. And so in order to serve as a pivot for the personal narrative – a name that seems to tie up all the narrative elements and close off new meanings – the subject position must be understood in terms of the significant forces of constitution that make up the bulk of the story. And so I have found it useful to include in conversations references to events and stories relating to many of the constitutive forces mentioned in previous chapters.

For example, my positioning discussions with Oscar included reference to parts of his subjectifying community, including the people (e.g., his ex-wife, his father, the dismissive salesman, himself, even me) whose actions positioned him as a failed man, and who in various ways reminded him of, and held him to that place. We spoke also of some of the ways in which he simultaneously complied with, as well as represented and recirculated, this discourse and its positioning of him. For instance, we discussed the expectation that he should, as a failed man, 'look down a lot and avoid eye contact' (in his words), and in other ways carry himself and present himself as a weak man. We discussed the ways in which his alternative presentations and knowledges of self were disqualified, such as when he began to feel empowered after 'speaking up', only to be shamed back into his more discursively appropriate place. We have seen in earlier chapters that all of these forces press down and hold the person to a problem-saturated identity. And so their entwinement in therapeutic discussions, and in our empathic understandings and reflections, adds weight to the constraints of the position itself.

Third, I want to emphasize the externalizing rather than internalizing quality of this kind of empathic engagement. On the one hand, the broad psychotherapy literature evidences a powerful and persuasive internalized reading of empathy, often conceptualized as the therapist's entering into something like the 'subjective inner world of the other' (Vanaerschot, 1990, p. 271). On such a reading, we understand the stories the person tells us in terms of the dynamics of the psyche or the person's internal, psychological world. Thus, Oscar's shame, his representations of his father and the mocking salesman, his temporary sense of empowerment when he spoke up, indeed his very sense of masculine ideals, might all be considered internal, psychological notions and expe-riences that must in some way be acknowledged, and allowed to come to some kind of order so that he can proceed onwards towards growth or self-actualization. His sense of himself as a failure might be read in terms of the ways in which his internal world is organized, and might be considered a sense or a belief which temporarily blocks his innate, internal tendency towards what Carl Rogers described as 'growth, matu-rity, and life enrichment' (Rogers and Sanford, 1989, p. 1491) – internal processes all.

But in narrative practice we take an externalizing view of these dynamics. We think of Oscar not as a self-contained unit, determined by his internal psychological dynamics, but as a perspectival point in a social and contextual drama. The book we are reading is not about Oscar's internal world, but his external one and his place within it. We have no direct access to that 'real' external world, however, except through our constructions, our stories of it. And so we listen to Oscar's stories about the world in which he lives; and we understand these sto-ries to be local, personally and contextually nuanced versions of those discourses and practices in the broader culture which have claimed him as one of their subjects. This means that Oscar's subject position – his sense of himself and of who he is – is not the internal centre of Oscar as such, but the central point of a particular story about his participation in that world. By virtue of his embodiment Oscar has no choice but to stand at the centre of the story that he tells. That is, as a constituted sub-ject with bodily form, he becomes the story's central perspectival point. Clearly, I am not saying that he stands at the centre of the cultural nar-rative or discourse, only that as an embodied being he is bound up at the storytelling centre of his own iteration and reiteration of those nar-ratives. He does not occupy any space other than the one provided by his corporeality, and so he can only speak and act from that point. His is the bodily place from which his story is told, heard, and felt. And all of this is roughly (though never fully) authored by the constituting forces of social practice and discourse.

Thus, the characters, plot lines, and other narrative components we hear about in Oscar's tellings are not to be thought of as referents to his 'psychology', but as elements of a narrative in performance; a narrative whose enactment relies on Oscar playing his part. Empathic positioning concerns itself with understanding what this 'part' is, with reference to, and in the context of, the broader constitutive social per-formance. This is a narrative whose integrity, coherence, and social performance in Oscar's life depends on his capacity to stand as its pivot, as its representative, and as its compliant subject. So we think of Oscar in a more or less centred position, placed there by a surrounding, external world of institutions, people, beliefs, and practices; not as the encapsulating 'psychological' whole within which his self-authored, solipsistic representations of these institutions, people, beliefs, and practices reside.

And finally, we should remember that the subject position anchoring the narrative is always a kind of caricature. It offers what is in some respects an absurd account, seizing upon a few interpreted elements of the person's existence and inflating them to ludicrous proportions. In a particular moment, it can resonate powerfully with the person's experience, leading to a kind of 'aha' moment. But almost immediately we see that the person cannot 'be' this position in its impossible one-dimensionality. Its experiential thickness belies its narrative simplicity and ultimate unsustainability. But as long as this narrative point is neither clarified nor fully inhabited – an inhabitation which can only but reveal its thinness – the person is vulnerable to remaining caught up in the discourses that implicate and hold him or her in that position. Indeed, the experiential depth of a problem-saturated position may rely to some extent on its fuzziness, because its narrative clarity has the potential to reveal its thinness, and its inability to offer a complete description of the person or of his or her life. So the person who is recruited into a problem-saturated position, which becomes known and precisely articulated, is well placed to prove and to even experience its status *as* caricature.

Moving towards ethics

Of course, this is not the end of the story. The person's capacity for resistance against limiting, caricaturizing identity conclusions is seldom sufficient, in itself, to allow him or her to move into different, preferred ways of being in the world. For that, we need to turn to an issue which I see as underpinning the whole narrative therapeutic exercise: ethics and ethical subjectivity.

7
From the Resisting Figure to the Ethical Subject

The prescriptions of discourse, boosted by its manifold mechanisms of subjection, require of its subjects a certain level of obedience to its normative declarations of what is right and what is wrong, of what is important and what is not. The constituted subject is inevitably a valuing subject.

For example, for Petra (who we met in Chapter 2), as romantic subject, what is valued above all else is an enduring romantic partnership. She is left cold by alternative formulations of what might be considered important, such as the notions of gender equality exemplified in Burr's (1995) critique of traditional practices of romance. Oscar, the man who feels a failure, values the tough masculine ideal he cannot attain. And Nobisa, a pregnant teenager in a family and a community of devout Christians, is pressed to value Christian morality, chastity, and her family's reputation in the community. It is evident that some of these persons' failures to attain the ideals set for them did not deter them from valuing those ideals nonetheless.

But resistance opens up the possibility not just of new positions, stories, and practices, but also other, often old, disqualified, hidden, or downgraded values, commitments, and principles: an alternative ethics. The person's resistances against imposed forms of selfhood bring him or her to 'the most intense point of a life, the point where its energy is concentrated' (Foucault, 2000a, p. 162). After all, at stake is one's very identity: 'Who must I be?', and also, 'Who can I become?' I have proposed that the human being is, by virtue of his or her embodied capacity for negative resistance, inherently equipped to offset the prescriptions that answer the first question. We often refuse, exceed, and spill over the confining dictates, 'you must be this; you must be that'. And while this resistance opens up the new question – 'who can I become now?' – it cannot, in itself, provide an answer.

Our corporeal excess flows nowhere in particular – it flows *away from* '*this*', but there is no a priori '*that*' to which it is oriented. It lacks its own narrative directedness. For example, Kevin's eventual revelation of the limits of the caricature position, 'I am a murderer' (see Chapter 6), exposes the fact that, in the end, he is not this. But it does not tell him who he can become. Resistance must be thickened through further storying activity. In this regard, I have found it useful to invoke Foucault's notions of ethical practice and the 'ethical subject' (Foucault, 1992, p. 27).

Moving from social constitution to ethics

For many authors, Foucault's late (e.g., 1992, 2001) turn to the issue of ethics, in his studies of ancient Roman and Greek civilizations, was confusing. His emphasis in these studies was not on how the Greeks or Romans were shaped by the forces of constitution into adopting certain ethical standards and practices – as one might have expected in the context of his earlier works – but on how individuals came to actively work on and inhabit their own ethical positions. We will discuss the meaning of 'ethics' below, but the point here is that Foucault had begun to describe how people were able to fashion their lives according to a certain style, ethos, or aesthetic, through various 'practices of the self' (Foucault, 1997d, p. 291). Michael White brought some of these ideas about what Foucault (1997c) also called the 'ethics of the self' (p. 255) into some of his reflections on narrative practice. For instance, in an interview with David Spellman he discussed his use of Foucault's schema for understanding ethical self-formation to construct questions for various therapeutic interviews (White, 2000, pp. 164–165).

But our enduring problem here has always been: how is this possible? The agentive ethical subject is here depicted – by both White and Foucault – as so much more active than Foucault's earlier constitutive writings on power/knowledge seemed to suggest was possible. And yet, Foucault never really put these two things together. Somehow, when he spoke about ethical self-formation, he seemed to ignore the question of power. And when he had earlier on spoken at length about power, the possibility of human agency and self-formation seemed unlikely. Indeed, White's use of Foucault traces this unevenness to some extent. He closely follows Foucault in developing an account of the constitutive effects of societal power dynamics and discourse, but, except for brief references to ethical self-formation, Foucault's name tends to disappear when White turns to issues of personal agency, intentionality, and preferred ways of living. Indeed, despite the significant influence of Foucault in earlier narrative texts and interviews, his name is hardly mentioned in White's (2007) final work, *Maps of Narrative Practice*; a work which powerfully emphasizes the agentive, intentional capacities of the person, and in which reference to Foucault is restricted to the notion of power as 'a mechanism of social control' (White, 2007, p. 268).

Of course, White is under no obligation to follow Foucault in each and every respect, but I wonder if narrative practitioners have taken to assuming – as Foucault's critics would have it – that Foucault is good for understanding power, but not so good for understanding personal agency. The more serious critique would be that narrative practice has inherited a kind of two-worlds theory: constitutive power/knowledge dynamics on the one side, and then, as if by magic, personal agency on the other. Two incompatible worlds cobbled together, allowed to coexist only on condition that their relationship is not examined too closely.

Indeed, the apparent discrepancy between personal agency and the forces of social constitution in Foucault's work led to various conclusions that he had, in the end, given up on his projects around power as a kind of lost cause, in favour of a more humanistic reading of the agentive human being. For instance, Žižek (2000) argues that Foucault is here attempting to 'break out of the vicious cycle of power and resistance', and 'resorts to the myth of a (human) state "before the Fall"' (p. 251); a reintroduction of the pristine, whole, pre-discursive human being, capable of self-determined action.

Foucault, some of his friends and peers, and many other scholars, vehemently oppose such readings (e.g., Deleuze, 1988; Veyne, 2010). But as I stated earlier, the point here is not to defend Foucault himself. Rather, our concern is that we can permit the retention of something like his power/knowledge formulation – something that matters a great deal to us in the field of narrative therapy – only on condition that it affords rather than negates some sense of personal agency. We are as committed to one as we are to the other, even as Žižek and others say they are irreconcilable. Thus, I tried to argue, especially in chapters 5 and 6, that something like an active, agentive being is already prefigured in the power/knowledge formulation: power can only work in the way that Foucault describes to the extent that persons are *already* active, corporeal beings, equipped with an inherent capacity for resistance, and hence personal agency. Indeed, I have argued that it is precisely power's recognition of this living, resisting being that leads it to be subtle, strategic, luring, and productive, rather than crass, brutish, threatening, and repressive. We noted in that discussion that Foucault did not go to great lengths to make this case himself, and perhaps he did not deliberately place such an active human being at the heart of his thought on power and discourse. What matters more than his intentions, though, is the fact that many subsequent scholars have since built a cogent argument that power relies upon, presupposes, and anticipates active, embodied, and agentive human capacity (e.g., Falzon, 1993; O'Leary, 2002).

On this understanding, the person who fashions his or her life in accordance with a certain style, ethos, or aesthetic (as Foucault found in the ancient Greeks and Romans), can be thought of not as a Foucauldian revision of the human being, but as precisely the multiple, embodied, resisting figure we discussed earlier, whose self-forming activities always take place within the context of power. This resisting figure, whose inherent multiplicity permits an overflowing of any constituted and finalized identity conclusions, can serve as an enabling platform for ethical self-fashioning. And at the same time, as I will argue below, the cultivation of an ethical subjectivity can entail an honouring of this being's refusal to be finalized, in a way that constituted subjectivity cannot.

But first, let me clarify what I mean by ethics.

What is ethics?

Broadly speaking, Foucault uses the notion of ethics to refer to the relationship the person has with him or herself, as opposed to the constitutive relationship the person has with knowledge or discourse. We will discuss in some detail below the ways in which this self–self relation can be thought to work, but for now let us note that the word 'ethics' refers to three interrelated aspects of existence.

The first is the conventional understanding of ethics as a sense of right and wrong. Our ethics give us a certain vision of how things should be, of how we should act, and of what we should stand for and against if we are to think of ourselves as ethical beings. However, it is important to note that the ethics with which we are concerned are of a personal nature; a morality 'with no claim to universality', says Veyne (1993, p. 2). When I speak of a person as embodying an ethical subjectivity, I am not thinking of his or her compliance with an already existing, universal, or rational set of ethical guidelines that we might find, for example, in various religious practices, or which flow from various scientific truths (as proposed, for example, by Skinner, 1953), or even in many of our professional ethics codes. Consequently, I do not think of ethics as a system of pre-scripted rights and wrongs which we might use to guide our therapy and our clients, such as is found in the work of Little and his colleagues (e.g., Little and Robinson, 1990), who attempt to rehabilitate criminal offenders by trying to instil certain predetermined moral values into their lives, or in the cognitive behavioural work of Callender (e.g., 1998), who in his 'moral suasion' therapy persuades clients to follow philosopher Immanuel Kant's ethical imperatives in their engagements with each other (e.g., in couples' therapy) or in their own lives (p. 274). The problem with such a priori determinations of what counts as ethics – whether proclaimed by a church, science, a professional organization, or a therapist's models – is that they involve impositions which control the person in socially constituted ways, and render him or her a docile, obedient subject. While we have seen that we often comply with such prescriptions, the ethical subject emerges in the spaces opened up by our unique ways of exceeding or resisting such impositions and their effects, enabling in turn a re-evaluation of our personal positions within the field of power and knowledge dynamics. So we are essentially talking about personal ethics, which incorporate a personal sense of rights and wrongs, about how things should be. The contents of this will be different for each individual, and granted nuance by his or her unique life experiences, forms of constitution, and the manner of his or her resistances.

The second aspect of ethics refers to that which, in a phrase used often by White, 'people ... accord value to in their lives' (e.g., 2006, p. 28). Ethics is not only about what people feel is right or wrong, but also about what is important to them. This might include special concerns people have, goals they have for living, beliefs they wish to uphold, principles they wish to honour, ideas which they are prepared to defend, and so on. For example, when I was a young boy my grandfather told me that he had made a decision to never intentionally hurt anybody. Of course, this might incorporate a sense of right and wrong, but it would be a mistake to conflate such a decision with the idea of a giant Superego wagging its finger at him, threatening guilt and shame should he not comply. My grandfather's emphasis was less on moralizing than it was on trying to honour something that was important to him. He had articulated a principle that he felt was valuable for both himself and the world in which he lived. So, here, ethical subjectivity includes that which is deemed valuable to and for the person.

The reader will notice that we are building a rather broad conception of ethics. But there is a reason for this breadth, which is to be found in the third, and perhaps most decisive aspect of ethics. This concerns Foucault's use of the term in its Greek manifestation: not exactly ethics, but 'ethos'. In *What Is Enlightenment*, Foucault (1997e) offers an insight into its meaning. Ethos is:

> a mode of relating to contemporary reality; a voluntary choice made by certain people; in the end, a way of thinking and feeling; a way too, of acting and behaving that at one and the same time marks a relation of belonging and presents itself as a task. (p. 309)

If ethics entails a 'mode of relating to contemporary reality', then clearly we are moving beyond our typical day-to-day usage of the term. It refers to a style, a determinate and distinctive way of being in the world, entailing a 'transformation of oneself for oneself' (Foucault, cited in Veyne, 2010, p. 105). Paul Veyne, using the term 'aestheticization' rather than 'ethos', says that Foucault was referring to something that stands as 'the opposite of (discursive) subjectivization' (2010, p. 105). This, Veyne says, is a personal 'initiative', in which the person takes himself or herself as 'the *oeuvre* upon which to work', who thereby gives himself or herself 'a morality...no longer upheld by God or tradition or reason' (pp. 104–107). But not just a morality; Foucault likens the idea of the self as an oeuvre to the relationship between an artist and his or her art. Thus, in response to our constitution in power and discourse dynamics, he says, 'we have to create ourselves as a work of art' (Foucault, 1997c, p. 262).

Foucault developed these ideas while studying ancient practices, but his intention was not for these studies to culminate in some kind of advice for us today. They cannot tell us which ethical forms to adopt – what kind of identity shape we should strive for – to best deal with the particular operations of power within whose context we live our lives. The modes of ethical self-formation used by the ancients would likely be irrelevant to us (Veyne, 2010). For Foucault, there can be no universal solution, or way of coping with, power. Our inevitable corporeal groundedness in our own, specific, historical eras (as discussed in Chapter 5) means that our tools for dealing with power must be fashioned in relation to, and out of, contemporary ways of knowing and doing. Consider that the ancient Greeks saw ethics as a practice of the aristocracy. We could no more use this vision of ethics to think through the kinds of racial, class, or gender discriminations with which we are concerned today, than we could use a hammer to retrieve lost data in a computer storage device. It simply doesn't fit in our context. The task of ethically working on oneself (as an oeuvre or work of art) must speak to the issues and practices of the day; indeed, to the issues and practices of each of our lives.

This is not to say that each person's ethics should be fully constituted by current social practices and beliefs; only that these ethics need to be in some way relevant to them, so that they can be meaningful to each person's particular existence. A personal ethos may include values, practices, principles, and beliefs, none of which are predetermined, but all of which are nevertheless to be found somewhere in the broader cultural horizon of meaning. They are not invented out of nothing. But we cannot prescribe what should count, for each individual, as ethical, valuable, or stylistic.

In sum, a personal ethos refers to principles which will have a bearing on one's sense of right and wrong, on what is accorded value in the person's life, and on the development of a *way* of conducting oneself, or a 'style of existence' (Veyne, 2010, p. 104) with its own unique form.

Who is the ethical subject?

The ethical subject is that person who has intentionally fashioned himself or herself in line with a particular ethos. This is a person who reconstitutes himself or herself, not as a subject of *knowledge*, but as a subject of *ethics*. While I will argue below that knowledge subjects (or constituted subjects) and ethical subjects differ in terms of their relationship to the person's embodied capacities for resistance, as well as to constitutive power dynamics in general, I should also say that ethics and knowledge are not mutually exclusive realms of life. In order to be a subject of ethics, one has to become subject to some way of *knowing* ethics in the first place. The ethical subject is, in other words, still a kind of constituted subject. What is perhaps more important about this distinction is that it refers to two ways of orienting to one's existence as a person.

On the one hand, the subject of knowledge poses for himself or herself the question: 'Who am I?' We have seen that for Foucault (e.g., 1990a), this is a culturally produced and historically specific question, which we are required to answer in some sense, in order not only to be socially recognizable and meaningful social partners, but also to be serviceable, to be useful, to power. The importance of this question, for Foucault, lies in its reflection of the fact that in the modern era we have come to place our highest value on knowing ourselves as individuals. Gros (2005) indicates that for us to ask this question of ourselves already demonstrates our obedience, in that the question is merely a personalized version of the question power, culture, society, demands we answer: 'Who are you?' We must answer, even if only by means of our names and addresses, so that society can 'know' and manage us; tax us; bill us; send us speeding fines; locate us in this or that nation, community, family, or school; decide if we are insiders or outsiders; hold us to the standards of our professions; track our movements over time; and so on. By making us individuals – specific individuals, belonging to this or that social category, with specific and knowable qualities, strengths, weaknesses, and disorders – society insures that we can be measured, assessed, compared against one another, and rendered subject to the various forms of normative judgements required to make modern power function properly. This is how we become useful and contribute to the reproduction of what is. Gros' point is that we obey by turning the societal requirement that we be identifiable, knowable individuals, into a personal quest that we set out to answer and to fulfil: 'Who am I?'

But our obedience goes further in that we do not decide for ourselves the answer to the question. Instead, we are told who we are. We are made into our selves. Before we even understand the question, our parents and caregivers, and the institutions and cultural practices into which we are recruited very early on, have already prescribed important parts of the answer. They provide us with a name, a language, and a birth certificate that proves that this – and nobody else – is who we are. They furnish us with rules and regulations regarding how we should move, dress, and speak, what we should like and not like, what we should aspire to, and what truths we should hold. They issue us with expectations structured by norms of gender, culture, religion, and so on. Platforms are thereby laid down, which fundamentally shape the future possibilities for our identities. And we have seen the terrific press on us to go on shaping our identities in some ways rather than others. In other words, our orientation to this question – 'Who am I?' – makes us susceptible to being installed as socially constituted subjects. This question, and the importance we put on it, contributes to our positioning as docile, compliant subjects, duly playing out our parts in a discursive performance whose terms, regulations, and prescriptions precede us.

On the other hand, the subject of ethics orients to a different kind of question: not 'Who am I?', but 'How shall I conduct myself? How shall I live my life?' One does not need to become pinned to a specific, recognizable identity in order to answer such a question. The ethical subject is one who has found a way to reflexively and intentionally identify with some socially available form of constitution and not others, and who has done so not out of obedience, habit, or tradition, but as a consequence of the cultivation of a personal ethos. Foucault seems to be suggesting that the privileging of ethics over knowledge might usefully dissolve the ossifying effects of the self-knowledge imperative.

The ethical subject derives its substance from a range of culturally available discourses, which, critically, can then be used to narratively and performatively thicken the person's resistances against those discourses which prescribe problem-saturated identities. In this regard, Foucault offers a cryptic, but telling statement: 'Equipment...is the medium through which logos is transformed into ethos' (in Rabinow, 2003, p. 1). Rabinow clarifies that by 'equipment', Foucault means the existing truths ('logoi') that circulate in the culture, and that it is through this knowledge-as-equipment (logos) that an ethos can be constructed. So we can only build answers to the ethical questions posed above by borrowing from existing knowledges (and so we recall White's and Foucault's insistence on the availability of social models for the fashioning of resistance). It is for this reason that Deleuze (1988) refers to such subjectivity as a 'fold' (p. 106); knowledges from the outside must be folded in order to produce something like an inside of subjectivity.

Inevitably, this will involve some degree of discursive compliance or adherence, insofar as the person follows the ethical (i.e., ethos inspired and inspiring) prescriptions with which he or she has identified, or – more cynically – into which he or she has been lured. But, from a post-structural Foucauldian perspective, this is an important kind of obedience because it serves as the very 'equipment' for our disobedience. The knowledge to which we intentionally, ethically, become obedient, must be part of what White (2004) describes as the 'materials lying about in society' (p. 103), which we can use to develop and thicken resistance. Once solidified in the person's life (an issue which I will discuss at length below), these discursively derived ethical commitments have the capacity to invest negative, embodied, but content-less resistances with meaning or content. In narrative terms, our ethical commitments give us stories, principles, values, and styles that allow us to do more than just 'say no' when our identities or life options are being closed down. They enable us to make something meaningful of our inherent overflowing multiplicity, in any particular instance. They thicken, rationalize, and enable a disciplined and more or less experientially coherent performance of resistance – in the name of a particular personal ethos – in the face of totalizing or otherwise objectionable practices. This readiness to

thicken resistance is associated with the ethical subject's ability to transfer his or her obedience (i.e., ethical commitments) into a range of life
contexts and emerging scenarios, by virtue of his or her enduring and
trans-contextual (though not infinite) identification with its principle,
its idea, its value, or its practice.

Thus, the ethical subject is one who is placed in a firm, side-taking,
and resistance-ready position within the broader context of the societal power dynamics in which he or she remains caught up. So if, as
Foucault (1992) tells us, 'power is everywhere' (p. 93) and unavoidable,
our ethical subjectivity gives us a place to stand within its machinations, and a developed justification for our resistances. We thereby avoid
being blown around by the winds of discourse, and take on what was so
important for Foucault, a degree of personal freedom.

The optimistic treatment I have given the concept of the ethical subject might well prompt the reader to wonder at this point: why did we
bother with all this talk of constitution when we have the notion of the
ethical subject to undo all that and paint a more hopeful picture? Have
narrative practitioners Zimmerman and Dickerson (1996) not already
told us that 'each of us can play a part in choosing what to let guide
us and in what contexts' (p. 93); that we are always already equipped
with the ability to 'choose' which discourses, which positions, which
power arrangements, and so on? Should we not simply have started
with that?

But we should consider that the ethical subject is a quite considerable
achievement in the face of what we have been made into; in the face
of the personal forms and social categories which have been imposed
on us. It is out of recognition of the achievement of ethical subjectivity
that Deleuze (1988) was led to say that the ancient Greeks 'invented'
the self–self relation that we call ethics (p. 102). On this account – and
it matters not whether we believe Deleuze's reading of history, only that
we hear how challenging a creation it was – the ethical subject is a strik-
ing accomplishment given its alleged emergence as a possibility for the
human being only after thousands of years of social living. So, conceptually, it is easy enough to say that we can counter our forms of
constitution through embodied resistances and the cultivation of some
form of ethical subjectivity; some kind of enduring, trans-situational
personal ethos. But we always have to do so in the face of power, running against the more or less coordinated flow of multiple forces telling
us who we are. How easy would it be for Oscar to simply *choose* another
way of being a man; or for Petra to simply choose values that were
not supportive of romance; or for Kevin to forgive himself following

the death of his friend? Zimmerman and Dickerson (1996) are right to suggest that there are always options, choices that can be made, but the reality is far more complex. And that is what I feel needs to be appreciated in order for us to develop a post-structural understanding of hope and personal agency. The forces of constitution stand as so many obstructions to our ability to step into our inherent multiplicity and to exercise the freedom Foucault says we already have.

The obstacles to adopting a personalized ethical self are multiple, and their articulation here might help us to appreciate what an achievement it is, or can be, as well as to understand the task that faces us as narrative practitioners. Let us remind ourselves of three such obstacles, which we have already come across in earlier chapters. First, power tends, via its representatives in families, institutions, and communities, to hold us to the identities it gives us. Indeed, it can exact powerful penalties, and often has the perceived right to effect rehabilitative operations on persons who deviate from its prescriptions. There are very real social forces which limit the degree to which we can exercise our freedom to be something other than what we have been made into. Second, the attainment of ethical subjectivity can involve 'refusing the self' (O'Leary, 2002, p. 107), and may therefore call upon us to go against something that feels inside us, part of us, inherently truthful, core to and an essential part of our being. And a third obstacle arises to the extent that values and ethical principles are rendered invisible *as values and ethical principles*. Instead, socially constituted values – those given to us – are often treated as truths, becoming background, taken-for-granted assumptions, even as they go on to shape our behaviour, thought, self-experience, ideals, and self-evaluations. The social construction of these values is invisible to the extent that they are naturalized, forming an invisible, boundaried horizon of meaning beyond which we cannot easily see. They seem beyond question.

It is in the face of such forces that an ethical subjectivity must be constructed.

Narrative practice and the ethical subject

In my view, narrative therapy offers a series of practices that seeks to meet and deal with these obstacles to the attainment of ethical subjectivity. This approach both relies on and enhances the person's capacity for a reflexive self–self relation such as I have described; one that entails an ability to capitalize on one's multiplicity and the overflowing of societal prescriptions by conducting oneself, in some measure, in accordance with a personal ethos or style, in accordance with what the person deems important, precious, or of value, and in accordance with some sense of what is right or wrong for him or her.

In this respect, let us consider White's (e.g., 2007) more recent work on intentionality as a means for conceptualizing personal agency. We can begin with his critical distinction between internal state and intentional state understandings. The former refers to understandings of 'human action as a surface manifestation of specific elements or essences of a self that is to be "found" at the centre of identity' (2007, p. 101). This may include ideas of intra-psychic processes, the unconscious, core beliefs, or a self-actualizing tendency as internal determinants of our actions. We have already discussed at length some of the problems with such internalizing views of the person. But White goes on to assert that these understandings, while not inherently 'wrong or invariably unhelpful', nevertheless '(d)iminish the sense of personal agency', isolate the person as if he or she were a self-contained rather than a relational being, and 'discourage diversity' in the sense that they rest on and reproduce norms for how persons should and should not be (pp. 104–105). On the other hand, he says, 'intentional state understandings of identity are distinguished by the notion of "personal agency"' (p. 103). Here, the person's intentions are seen to lend a kind of directionality to his or her conduct, thought, manner of being in relationship, and broader experience. For White, narrative conversations drift towards intentional rather than internal state understandings, because the former enable the realization of a more active, agentive stance in ways that the latter cannot.

How does one access intentional state understandings? I do not want to discuss this in too much detail, lest we lose focus (the interested reader can consult White, 2007, pp. 75–128), but in summary we can say that this involves a movement, in therapeutic conversations, from what is described as the 'landscape of action' towards the 'landscape of identity' (White, 2007, pp. 78–81). As the person tells his or her story, he or she often talks about actions, happenings, and events in his or her life. This is the landscape of action. The therapist listens to these tellings, and pays close attention to any special, unique, or agentive moments embedded in them; perhaps there are hints of the person's resistance, or some out-of-phase development or initiative. The person is then encouraged to reflect on the meaning of these unique outcomes, and on the intentions, beliefs, values, purposes, principles for living, and commitments reflected in them. These reflections entail a move towards the landscape of identity, insofar as they build a sense, not of the story or events as such, but of the person as agent within them (see also Carey and Russel, 2003). The practitioner zigzags between these two landscapes, with stories of actions and events providing a personal and historical ground for the values, purposes, and principles that are identified, insuring that the latter are always experience-near, and linked to the person's concrete, corporeal life as it has been lived. Invariably, these conversations privilege the values or principles that the person stands for, represents, or in other ways orients to. When the person speaks about preferred outcomes or developments, he or she is inevitably talking about things that have value for him or her.

The therapist might ask about these in many different ways. For instance, in one session, White meets with 15-year-old Liam, whose mother is concerned that he feels 'messed up' and 'paralyzed in life' (p. 89). In consultation with Liam, White sees this as the dominant, problem-saturated storyline. Intertwined with conversations about actions, White asks questions that move talk towards the landscape of identity. He asks Liam questions about 'what was precious' to him (p. 84), 'what this (action) reflects in terms of (his) values' (p. 87), 'where (he) stands' (p. 91), 'what's important' to him (p. 91), what he is 'aspiring to' (p. 92), what he has 'held onto' (p. 93), and what his 'purposes' are. What are these questions aimed at, if not the very ethical subject of which we are speaking?

It is no surprise then, that the dialogue generates personally meaningful, ethically flavoured concepts. In this case, notions of 'fairness' and 'salvaging life' – gleaned from various actions, including Liam's distracting of his abusive father to help his mother – stand out as meaningful to Liam. The thickening of these concepts assists in his movement away from a sense of being messed up and paralysed, and towards an identification with a different kind of self-story. But this is a self-story that is decidedly ethical rather than knowing in its tone; it orients more to the question 'How shall I live?' than the typically prescribed, finalizing question 'Who am I?' The values that emerge in the conversation (fairness and salvaging life) denote the emergence of an ethical subjectivity insofar as they can be used to point, in a highly personalized way, to the three aspects of ethics we discussed earlier: as references to right or wrong actions (e.g., fairness is right for Liam, unfairness is not); as indicators of what is important to Liam as he deals with life's challenges; but also as emblems of a broader style or way of being in the world, which might not yet be articulable, but which might still emerge as these two concepts find real-world application. As new and unexpected situations arise, the application of 'salvaging life', for instance, might take on nuanced meanings, link up with other values and stories to form new concepts, or come in some other way to be re-interpreted.

In other words, through re-authoring, a certain style of living and engaging with the world begins to be articulated, and Liam seems to identify with the concepts that give this ethos narrative intelligibility and substance. To be clear, these named contents of a style of life are not invented by Liam – fairness and salvaging life are ideas that already exist in the broader culture – but because we can be nothing without some kind of disciplined social constitution (c.f., Smith, p. 149), these are (for now) the principles he identifies with, which he can use to intentionally shape his conduct, and through which he can become something other than what he was. This is partly achieved via his ability to identify, in conversation with his mother and his therapist, an initially sketchy, but increasingly thickened personal history. It is not that he 'is' fair, or a salvager of life. It is more a case of these notions resonating with certain aspects of his life, such that he is able to *intentionally* identify with and orient to them as a way of crafting a life.

What strikes me here is that the person's answering of the kinds of questions that the narrative therapist asks moves that person not only from the landscape of action to that of identity, not only from internal to intentional frames of reference, but also from constituted subjectivity to something approximating ethical subjectivity: 'I am messed up and paralysed in life' becomes 'I value fairness and the salvaging of life'. Narrative conversations frequently move, albeit not in some many words, from the question of self-knowledge – who am I? – towards the question of ethical subjectivity – how shall I run my life? After all, in narrative practice the person is seen as a socially constituted figure, but with a pre-existing capacity for resistance as well as for reflexive self–self engagement, which is to say, an ethical subjectivity. I find it useful to think of these therapeutic practices as capitalizing on these capacities and providing conversational means for their thickening. These conversations contribute to the sourcing of some of the 'equipment' that Foucault said is needed to transform logos into ethos; to move from self-knowledge into preferred ways of being in the world.

A case

I would like to outline some of my work with a 28-year-old man, who experienced anxiety and panic attacks in the context of a difficult work situation. I will use this case, together with White's work with Liam, to point to some of the main features of the ethical subject, and to discuss ways in which ethical subjectivity can be narratively and experientially thickened.

Carl was a single man, who lived alone in a small apartment, a few minutes' drive away from his parents, to whom he said he was still close. In the first few minutes of our meeting, he spoke about his panic attacks and 'obsessions', which he interpreted to mean that he was not 'very tough'. He berated himself for being so 'fragile, like a delicate little China doll' that he had to take anti-anxiety medications for 'a little bit of work stress'. I thought this was a rather tough self-assessment. I asked him to tell me about his work stress. Carl told me that he worked in an engineering company, and that he was greatly distressed about some interpersonal issues that had come up at work. He felt he was being treated with considerable disrespect by a colleague, Zeph. This treatment had him so upset that he found himself 'obsessing' about it, and losing sleep, which in turn made his work days even more difficult to get through. He told me that when he started working at the firm a year before, he and Zeph got on quite well. However, after a few months, Carl was surprised to be summoned to his boss' office, after Zeph had complained that Carl was 'nowhere to be found' when a client arrived. Zeph had complained further that he had to rescue the situation by meeting with this client, which not only interfered with his own duties, but caused embarrassment because he did not know this particular client's situation. Carl told me it was true that he had left the office for 15 minutes at that time. However, the context of this was that he had offered to do a favour for Zeph, helping one of his friends in another part of the building; and besides, the client was not expected and had arrived without an appointment. Carl described feeling betrayed and set up, and while his boss did not come down on him too hard, he was worried about being marked as unreliable so early on in the job.

The relationship between Carl and Zeph deteriorated after that. For instance, one day he overheard Zeph saying demeaning things about him to two work colleagues, and they ended up laughing at Carl's expense. When Carl eventually walked into the room, making his presence known, Zeph and the others immediately changed the subject. They even greeted him with a smile. Carl tried to pretend he had not overheard their conversation, because he was unsure how to handle the situation. He told me that even though he had a feeling Zeph was saying bad things about him behind his back, this was the first confirmation of this, and it had still come as a shock. The fact that others had joined in was especially distressing. In response to all of this, and despite his sense of himself as a friendly, warm person, Carl had become withdrawn at work, and did not join his colleagues when they got together for lunches or for casual social events after work.

I asked Carl what he thought was going on. He said that he was confused, and had no idea why Zeph had gradually turned on him, or why he had begun to poison others' impressions of him. Carl said that he had not had much experience with 'people like this', and that he wasn't up for 'such a cutthroat work environment'. I asked him to tell me a little more about his limited experiences of 'people like this'. Because our stories about others often implicate self-positioning, I hoped this discussion would move us closer towards the position Carl occupied. As argued above, it can be helpful to identify persons' problem-saturated subject positions, as a way of acknowledging their situation and meeting them in the form of 'who they are' in that moment, but also as a way of seeking out the finalizing identity conclusions that reside at the heart of their narratives. So the question in my mind was something like, 'who are *you* in relation to "people like this"?' Further examples of his interactions with 'such' people might help clarify both our understandings of this.

He told me that when he was 14 years old, he had a friend who was being bullied. Carl initially said and did nothing about this, and admitted that he had been scared and intimidated. He stood by while his friend suffered. But one day, when the bullying started up again, Carl intervened. He told me, laughing, 'before I even knew it, I was shouting at this massive guy and I told him to pick on someone his own size'. The bigger boy laughed at him, but, to Carl's relief, walked off. Evidently, this bigger boy was an example of the 'people like this' that Carl had spoken about when thinking of Zeph.

Of course, I am alert to the conversational possibilities afforded by Carl's action, as a 14-year-old boy, of telling off the bully confronting his friend; it could stand as a unique outcome and help bring forth different ways of thinking and doing. But in the moment, I had two other more pressing concerns. First, in that moment I felt that Carl was still preoccupied with his current situation, and I had the sense that his talk of earlier experiences of 'people like this', while interesting, had diverted him somewhat. And second, we had not yet clarified precisely in which ways the childhood situation was relevant to his current circumstances.

I noticed that Carl had not yet used the word 'bully' or 'victim' in relation to his current situation, but he had used these terms freely when recalling the situation with his friend some 14 years earlier. These were his words, which I assumed had some relevance to our discussion about 'people like' Zeph. I took this as a kind of permission to introduce these notions into his current context. My interest was not so much in exploring why there was this difference (why he had not used these words in relation to his current context). I am not trying to identify any denials or other psychic defensive manoeuvres. Rather, at this point I am merely trying to find a way to articulate Carl's subject position, using the terms of the narrative framework he was working in. I would leave it to him to decide whether or not a particular phrase or word (such as 'bully' or 'victim') made sense.

I decided to put what I was hearing into words: 'What I understand from what you are saying is that when you were 14 you were afraid and intimidated by the bully who was bullying your friend, but now you are the one who is being bullied.' Carl stumbled for words in response, and I wondered if I had put it too strongly: 'Or if the word "bullied" sounds wrong', I said, 'it could be the wrong word here ... ' He sighed and said it was 'the right word'. It seemed I was on the right track, and that we were in the proximity of his central position in this particular narrative, so I went on:

> So if I understand then, you're intimidated, you're afraid, you're powerless, and you're alone. To make it worse, you're a fragile, delicate China doll. You're so intimidated and fragile that you can't even spend time with the people you work with anymore. Okay, some part of you tells you to socialise with them. But how can you do that, how is that possible now? Of course you can't. You're a victim, you're too brittle and fragile to just hang out! (four-second pause) I don't know Carl, that's what I hear, does that come close to what this is like?

Carl stared at me for a time, and eventually said, 'Yeah, you hit the nail on the head'. It seemed to me that we had found a rather precise narrative point, which had powerful resonance for Carl, despite his apparent discomfort with it. We had found words to talk about his stuckness in a particular subject position from which he wanted to escape, but could not yet find a way out of.

Carl returned to see me two weeks later, and spoke about needing to 'tackle this bullying nonsense again', just as he had done as a 14-year-old boy. It seemed to me that the naming of his position, in as clear and distinct a way as we could, had contributed to a making visible of his capacity to exceed and overspill the finalizing, restrictive truth of his positioning as a scared, powerless, and fragile victim. His reference to his situation as a kind of 'nonsense' to be 'tackled' sounded to me like a kind of disobedience, which effectively loosened the grip of the problem-saturated discourse that had rendered him its subject. To use Klossowski's (2005) metaphor, the equilibrium of the power-subject relationship was destabilized, and Carl was able to gain a brief but potentially significant ascendancy. And so a therapeutic opportunity presents itself: we both see that the negative identity conclusion we had arrived at does not do Carl justice, and it cannot fully explain who he is. To take advantage of this implicit recognition, and given his declared intention to 'tackle this bullying nonsense again', I wondered if a conversation about how he had handled the bully when he was 14 might offer us the beginnings of a pathway that led away from the problem-saturated identity conclusions we had come to, but which had been found wanting. After all, his resistance against the negative identity conclusion we had reached does not provide guidance on what he should do, but only impels him to do *something*. So we were in need of some narrative direction. His actions against the bigger boy who was intimidating his friend interested me in this respect, because they signalled something different than his sense of being a victim, and something other than China-doll fragility.

So I asked Carl to explain why he had taken the risky decision to stand up to the bully so many years ago. He corrected me, and told me it was not really a decision, but a 'spur of the moment' thing. But then he said he remembered as a young boy being excited by the Shakespeare play, *Hamlet*, which he had studied in school. A particular line from that play stood out for him, which he remembered as 'something about to be true to yourself'. He said it's not that he was intentionally being 'true' to himself by standing up to this bully, but that in the end he did feel he had been honest to himself and how he was feeling. It fitted also, he said, with his father's approach to the world, which involved, from Carl's perspective, being honest, and speaking up even when it was uncomfortable to do so. Carl greatly admired this quality of his father's, and guessed that it had something to do with why this Shakespearean phrase (as he recalled it) stood out for him. It seemed to connect him to his father.

Since I am wary of staying with some essential notion of a 'self' to which Carl must be true, I asked him what it was that he was being true to in his actions in that schoolyard bullying situation. That is, as White (2007) suggests, rather than staying with some 'internal' understanding of who he actually 'is' (the self to which he is true), I sought to move towards an 'intentional' understanding of what he values and what he can intentionally perform. We struggled with this question for a while, and I told him about other questions I was thinking about, like: 'How could you recognize when you were being true to yourself?'; 'Is there any way I would know, as an observer?'; 'How do you think your friend made sense of your actions? And the bully?' We mulled over these questions, and Carl concluded that being true to himself was 'something to do with speaking up even when it was difficult, like speaking up against bullying and intimidation and abuse'. He went on: 'It reminds me of something like "truth to power". I'm not sure exactly what that means, but it's that sort of thing.'

Turning back to his current situation, I asked if his reflections on these things – and I listed them: the Shakespeare phrase; his father's moral courage; his being true to the value he had placed on speaking up; the personal resonance of the idea of truth to power – might assist in his decision to tackle 'this bullying nonsense' at work. He seemed energized by this idea, sat forward in his chair, clasped his hands together, and looked out the window, as he said, 'Yes, absolutely'. Carl then told me that, until our discussion, he had forgotten all about the Shakespeare quote, and how meaningful it had been for him as a child. I asked him if he was interested in reconnecting with the idea and its personal meaning for him, and he said he was. He agreed with my guess that these memories – of reading Shakespeare, of his dealing with the childhood bully, and of his appreciation of his father's ways of being – could be useful starting points for such a reconnection, and I asked him if he had any ideas on how else he might strengthen this connection. In response, Carl seemed to have an 'aha' moment: 'I'll look it up!' 'What do you mean?' I asked. He said: 'I want to look up the actual phrase Shakespeare used. It's rusty in my memory. I want to find it again.'

This seemed a wonderful idea. It was not that I had any special knowledge of what Shakespeare meant, or that I thought the actual quote contained nuanced meanings that could add to his sense of it. But I thought that the very act of trying to locate and study the phrase might facilitate and concentrate his intentionality around this. It might help ground his emerging ethical subjectivity in the landscape of action; in the world of corporeal, lived action. This move to find the Shakespeare quote signalled the beginning of Carl's active reconnection with a long-forgotten personal project, which had as its central point his principled decision to be 'true' to himself.

In our third session, before turning to the Shakespeare quote, I asked Carl about his work situation. He told me he had felt compelled, despite extreme anxiety, to speak openly with Zeph. He scheduled a formal meeting and expressed his sadness and disappointment that Zeph had taken to unfair bullying tactics, by misrepresenting him to their boss and to their colleagues, and which, he told Zeph, had left him in a vulnerable, exposed, and isolated position. Zeph defended himself, saying Carl had the wrong end of the stick, and accused him of being 'oversensitive'. While relating this, Carl told me he'd come to the realization that Zeph would not accept what he had done, and that there was little that could be done to change that. Nevertheless, he said he came away from that meeting trembling, but also with a sense of 'fullness', a kind of 'fulfilling feeling', that he was being 'true' to himself, even if (he felt) Zeph could not be honest about what had happened.

At that point, I smiled at Carl and said, 'Go on, tell me, did you find the quote?' Carl bent over, reached into his satchel, and brought out a battered old brown book. He explained that he decided he didn't want to look up the phrase on the internet, but to find the original Shakespeare book he had used when he was at school. A few hours after our last session, he had visited his parents' house and went through their attic. After quite a search, he found the book. He opened it to where he had inserted a bookmark, and showed me his 14-year-old pencil marks, circled around the quote, which read:

> This above all: to thine own self be true,
> And it must follow, as the night the day,
> Thou canst not then be false to any man.

These actions and reflections did not entirely remove the stress of his work situation, but they were useful in affording him an ethical platform from which to engage with the fields of power swarming around him.

There is far more to tell about my work with Carl, and I will come to some of that below. But for now, let us pause to consider some of the more formal aspects of the ethical subject, with reference to the personal project Carl was embarking on, to White's work with Liam, and to therapeutic work more generally.

Thickening the ethical subject in practice

I would like to propose four interrelated ideas to aid in the therapeutic development of a thickened account of the ethical subject: first, the ethical subject involves an alignment of principles and conduct; second, it requires some degree of focused intentionality; third, the form of one's ethical subjectivity must be buttressed for it to remain viable and usable over time and across contexts; and fourth, it situates the person as an active participant in what Foucault (1997d) called society's 'games of power' (p. 299).

These considerations emerge from Foucault's writings and lectures, on life in Ancient Greece and Rome in particular (e.g., Foucault, 1990b, 1997d, 2001), and various interpretations of those works (e.g., Gros, 2005; Veyne, 1993). Let us consider each in turn.

The alignment of principles and conduct

In narrative therapy, dialogue orients more around the question 'How shall I conduct myself?' than 'Who am I?' Indeed, many sub-questions of the former frequently arise in re-authoring, re-membering, and unique outcome conversations. In the process, the person begins to articulate some principle or principles around which to organize his or her conduct. For example, we saw in the case White (2007) describes that Liam is able to identify with the notions of 'salvaging life' and 'fairness'. These are notions that resonate with his sense of what was important to him (in the landscape of identity) when reflecting on how he had conducted himself at various significant points in his life (in the landscape of action). I have argued that this is not a unique feature of this particular case, but that very often in narrative therapy some such principles – indicators of what is of value to the person – are rendered salient, serving to anchor his or her commitments and practices, and stand as a kind of guiding thread for the conversation. We saw also in my work with Carl, that we were able to identify his valuing of 'speaking up even when it is difficult'; an idea that had been valuable and important to him in his younger years, and which he was able to reconnect with now as an adult, in thinking about how he might conduct his life in the face of challenging circumstances. The articulation and storying of these principles or values can be useful in affording the person a sense of purpose and meaning not only as he or she goes about his or her life, but also in the difficult contexts in which he or she is interpellated into a problem-saturated identity.

The success of this endeavour rests on the person's ability to align principles on the one hand, with conduct on the other. So this is the first point I wish to make about the relationship between conduct and principle, which is summed up well by Gros (2005), who, commenting on Foucault's studies of ancient Greek and Roman civilizations, notes the importance of the question: 'Do my actions today correspond to the principles that I have given myself?' (p. 703).

The second point about the relationship between principle and conduct is a reiteration: I do not think of these principles as located within the person's psyche. Rather, they are culturally shaped ideas, beliefs, and practices, out there in the world of social happenings, which become appealing and meaningful to particular individuals, in particular ways, and which come to have centripetal effects on the person's awareness in particular moments (and sometimes, over more extended time periods). Thus, my attempt to honour Carl's notion of 'being true to oneself' does not require my belief that there is some inner, essential self to which he is true. Nevertheless, this is a potentially essentializing notion, and so the conversation moves to the living principles to which it gives way in his case: 'speaking up when it is difficult' and 'speaking truth to power'. But I do not think of these in terms of Carl's supposedly 'true self'. He is not, in essence, a defender of justice or an opponent of bullying. Rather, as White and Foucault have already told us, these are ideas lying about him, some of which have been forgotten for reasons we do not understand. They are cultural artefacts which he rediscovers, picks up, dusts off, and polishes (the Shakespeare book is quite literally dusted off and read), and around which he begins to circle in an increasingly complex, but nevertheless disciplined series of movements. But it is a dance with which he has some familiarity: he witnessed his father's performance of some of its moves, he confronted the boy bullying his friend, and he recalls the moving effects of the words of Shakespeare on his 14-year-old self, which remind him of the values that matter to him: not to be 'himself', precisely, but to speak up, even when it is difficult to do so.

This brings us to the third point about principle–conduct alignment. The meanings of these principles become unique to the lives and circumstances of the persons who identify with them. The manner of their performance is, in other words, not restrained to singular, dictionary-like definitions, but is always context-specific and prone to spontaneous and unpredictable diversification. Despite the wide availability and common usage of articulated principles like fairness, speaking up, and salvaging life, their meanings are inevitably shaped according to the unique histories, perspectives, and emergent circumstances of the people who find value in them. We would surely all agree with Liam that something like fairness is a good thing; but this does not mean that we understand it in the way that he does. The widespread availability and support of this principle does not at all point to a universal understanding of what it means in practice. Indeed, a commitment to fairness might prompt two parties to go to war with each other, precisely because their understandings of what fairness means are not the same, but are shaped by their respective histories, conditions of living, religious and cultural practices and beliefs, and so on. Thus, the manner in which conduct aligns with principle will necessarily be shaped by local contextual and personal factors, and in terms of each person's lived and embodied experience. In addition, the meaning of a given principle in a person's life is subject to change. After all, our corporeal existence in a dynamic material world requires us – and our principles, our ethics – to be responsive to contingent circumstances. Our principles inevitably get caught up in and shaped by the hustle and bustle of the social worlds in which we live. Our bodily grounding insures that a given principle never stays in some pristine, idealized form, because it must be adapted, twisted, bifurcated, rethought, and applied in novel ways as life happens around us. Initially, in our discussions about Carl's interest in speaking up against bullying and power, we have a specific set of circumstances in mind, which enables a more or less precise pinning down of what it means right here and now. But then, when life moves on, we notice that the principle's ongoing relevance will to some extent depend on its elasticity and adaptability. I could not have predicted, for instance, how this principle would proliferate in unique ways in Carl's life: that speaking up would include letting a restaurant manager know when his food was poorly prepared; or telling a woman that he had feelings for her, despite others' warnings that it was 'too soon' to say such things.

The reader might wonder, as some of my psychoanalytic colleagues have asked, whether it is somewhat artificial to think of personal change in terms of intentionally orienting to some principle or value. But we should remember that we are all, in a sense, very well practised in doing precisely that. We have already been socially constituted, and live our lives as subjects; as figures who typically obediently align our conduct with particular discursive expectations and requirements. But Foucault and Deleuze have shown that unlike such social forms of constitution, a stable and enduring ethical self–self relation does not come easily. This is a task and a practice of intentionally and purposefully giving ourselves, rather than having imposed upon us, certain principles to follow, even in the most difficult of circumstances. Considerable work is required for it to become habitual, to come to feel, experientially, part of who we are. This is why, in narrative practice, the witnessing of resistance, and the identification of unique outcomes, the absent but implicit, and even of values and principles for living, are not typically in themselves sufficient to enable the person to move decisively away from problem-saturated identities.

But their identification, and their conversational link with conduct (in the landscape of action) represents an important step in the journey of building an ethical subjectivity, the attainment of which grants persons a sense of personal agency, a clear place from which to speak or act, and thereby 'a relation of belonging', as Foucault (1997e, p. 309) describes it: a belonging to a definite set of principles, and, by virtue of its inevitable side-taking effects, a belonging to a certain community of social actors, and sometimes to certain social causes rather than others. But the ethical subject must be constructed, built, trained, and practised if these effects are to be realized. So it is with this question in mind that I move now to touch on a useful step to take after the naming of these principles: the assumption of the right kind of intentionality.

Intentionality and athletic concentration

How does the person become what Veyne (1993) calls 'the patriot of his or her own values' (p. 3)?

The ethical subject's capacity to stay attuned to given principles rests on an ability to recognize and make use of spaces or situations for their enactment and performance. This involves an intentional focus, at least to start with, such that the person actively interprets situations in which the performances of these principles would be appropriate and useful. The active dimension of this intentionality is not to be underestimated. Consider the assumption, still found in many therapies, that 'an individual's behaviour is in some way due to a lack of awareness of his or her motivations underlying it' (Scaturo, 2010, p. 823). Such understandings may promote the idea that the cultivation of self-awareness, or insight into the truth of one's internal being, leads to change (we should note, however, that many psychoanalytic and humanistic practitioners no longer make such a simplistic assumption; but such a view still circulates and I want to use it to highlight some of the distinct features of the promotion of ethical subjectivity in therapeutic practice). For those of us in the post-structural narrative tradition, the ethical subject is not a figure of introspection and inward reflection who, having identified a particular, personally resonant principle is content to contemplate its meaning and allow it to unfold in its own time and in its own fashion; as if springing from an internal well that had just been tapped. Clearly, we should not think of the naming of a principle – fairness, standing up to bullying – as a kind of insight, releasing the energy of some repressed, stored-up truth so that it can go on to be naturally expressed. Instead, the principle needs to be put to work, under the guiding hand of intentionality.

In this regard, Gros (2005) thinks of the ethical subject as requiring a kind of 'athletic concentration' (p. 701). So, in contrast to the therapeutic posture of promoting inward reflection to enable insight and a release of the forces of change, here we think of ethical subjectivity as a work, requiring focus, training, practice, and *action*. Because the ethical subject is a figure of action, our focus is on what he or she will *do* with his or her ethics. In his studies of ancient practices, Foucault (2001) noted various practices of the self that convey a sense of this active intentionality, including 'techniques of meditation, of memorisation of the past, of examination of conscience, of checking representations which appear in the mind, and so on' (p. 11). These are training techniques that discipline the person for future ethical conduct.

In our own therapeutic practices, the intentional deployment of a principle in the landscape of action can occur in many ways. We see this, for example, in the therapist's encouragement of the person to think forward to what a particular value or principle 'makes possible' in his or her life. Narrative practitioners frequently want to know how certain realizations of principles, commitments, or aspects of life accorded value will be put to use. For instance, White's (2007) re-authoring conversations with Liam promote the visibility of certain actions that Liam can take to intentionally maintain the link between conduct and principle into the future. These future performances are – by virtue of the re-authoring conversation's identification of their previous manifestations – lent support by analogous performances in the past. Re-authoring shows Liam that he has, in his own personal history, been *trained* in these performances to some degree. This makes them more possible in the future.

Let us take, for example, Jill Freedman's detailed account of her discussions with a woman, Hollie, who has been influenced by cultural models that stipulate that women should tolerate unpleasant situations and not have too loud a voice (Freedman and Combs, 1996). In the conversation, Hollie comes to the realization that such cultural models led her to suppress her voice, and not to heed the trust she had in herself. Now, she makes a significant decision: 'when I feel something, . . . I really have to act on it, instead of suppressing it' (p. 166). Ethics compel action – therein lies their potential for personal agency – and so Hollie experiences a compulsion to align her conduct with the newly articulated principles concerning trusting her voice. Freedman then asks some questions to clarify, and to discover what this might make possible: 'So what do you think will be the next thing that will happen with this to move it into different aspects of your life?' (p. 167). And then, 'What would be an example of something that maybe you wouldn't have done five years ago, that you think you might begin to do now in one of those other contexts?' (p. 167). And again: 'Okay. So, it will be interesting to see … where this leads' (p. 168). Freedman strongly focuses the conversation on what Hollie's realization makes possible into the future, into different contexts, precisely because she recognizes that this realization is not an *insight* that leads inexorably to its own positive changes, but refers to a principle that must be intentionally inserted into life, put to work, adapted, serviced, and rehearsed, in order for it to be usable, relevant, and productive in the real world that Hollie lives in.

We can also consider Carl's spontaneous decision to seek out his dusty old schoolbook, which contained the quote he was looking for, as an example of such an intentional approach. His search is an active performance, out there in the world, and I see it as part of our jobs to support this. We had explored some of the historical situations in Carl's life in which the values that mattered to him were enacted. And then, looking to the future, I asked Carl what he would do with this book now that he had found it, in what other circumstances he might find its message relevant, and how he might remember its meaning for him, and its historical resonance. Indeed, I have found some simple questions to be useful in fostering such intentionality: 'How will you remember this?'; 'What stories from your life do you need to remind yourself of?'; 'What should you put in your pocket and bring with you when you go into that meeting, to keep you focused on your intentions?'; 'Who might help you remember?'; 'In what circumstances might you be pressed to forget this?'

I recall one set of conversations with another young man who, going against all family expectations, decided to give up on his high-paying job, and go travelling so that he could re-assess his life. The problem he now faced was how to tell his father, who he found to be an intimidating and conservative figure who would almost certainly disapprove of his decision. He was not sure how to prepare for this meeting, and feared he would give in to his father's pressures. In our previous discussions, we had identified integrity and honesty as important values for him, and we spoke about several examples of his performance of these values at different points in his life. These past performances could now be seen as rehearsals, a certain kind of training, for his participation in future events. So together we explored the questions of whether these values would be useful in his interaction with his father, and then of how he could remind himself of them as he built up to that meeting. He decided that before meeting his father he would put in his pocket a copy of a letter he had written to his boss, in which he had expressed with honesty and integrity his concerns about the way the organization was being run: one of the previous iterations of this kind of performance. This document would serve as a tangible reminder of the value he placed on integrity and honesty, a value in which he had already had some training, such that at any point in the conversation with his father he could reach into his pocket, feel the texture of those pages, and refocus his intentions (see Guilfoyle, 2011).

In such ways, persons can be supported in going into difficult situations with an intentional, athletically focused approach, having become aware of the historical ways in which they have already performed their ethical commitments, enabling them in turn to enact those principles into the future.

An ethically fortified subject

Gros (2005) makes the point that the ethical subject is a 'strong subject', characterized by his or her 'ethical fortification' (p. 701). The significance of this with respect to our previous discussions is that a fortified subject is one who can stand with some surety and resilience within the constitutive fields of power and discourse practices. Through the person's development of a kind of mastery relative to the principles with which he or she is aligned – a mastery which may be fostered by thickened personal narratives as well as by a supportive community – the ethical subject is able to take and maintain a position relative to such forces; although always from within, never from the outside of power. We can contrast this with the stark image of the person who is 'blown by the wind and open to the external world...someone who lets all the representations from the outside world into his mind' and 'accepts these representations without examining them, without knowing how to examine what they represent' (Foucault, 2001, p. 131). This is a figure who can find no personal bearings or ethical platform, and is at the whim of the forces of social alignment which seek to capture and put him or her to use in their service. While this hypothetical figure is empirically unlikely, it does offer us a useful image against which to consider the ethically fortified subject.

In my view, re-authoring, re-membering, outsider witness, and definitional ceremony practices (e.g., White, 2000, 2007) are powerful narrative technologies for the promotion of fortified ethical subjectivity. These practices serve to ground preferred identities, and the values and principles that support them in the person's life (in the past, present, and future), and also to locate these developments in a social context which has the potential to lend further support for their ongoing performance.

Recall that in my work with Carl, for instance, it emerged that his father stood out for him as someone who was 'true' to himself even in the face of difficulty. And so we spoke about how his father might respond to some of the developments in Carl's life, such as his decision to take a stand against bullying and to speak up even when it was uncomfortable. We also spoke about how it might be for his father to hear how he had inspired Carl. Carl decided to speak to his father about the steps he was taking, and about how his favourite Shakespeare quote reminded him of him. He told me later that his father was very touched, and said that it was no surprise to him that his son would take such a stand. He told Carl about certain memories he had of Carl that reminded him of this ability. For example, he remembered Carl at around the age of four becoming upset when he saw a television programme in which a man was verbally abusive towards a woman. Carl did not even remember some of these events, but their narration helped further ground his sense that he was indeed well prepared to engage in the project of living according to the ethical standards he had identified.

As this example suggests, the principled strivings of the ethical subject are not only bolstered by their identification, their intentional deployment, and their re-authoring. Foucault makes it clear that there is a vital, even constitutive, social component to the formation of ethical subjectivity, such that it is never a purely individual project. Given the person's inevitable situation in the social field of power/knowledge dynamics, his or her ethically inspired actions are always fundamentally relational (and, as we shall see below, political) in nature. After all, we have seen that the ethical subject is always already yet another, albeit preferred, kind of constitution or form of subjection; its form and its components are always to be found in the culture that surrounds us. In a sense, it is relational in its very inception. We will see below, too, that it has relational effects in the context of power. But it is relational also in its maintenance. The move towards ethical fortification is enhanced to the extent that it is, at least in some minimal ways, supported or afforded (which is not to say it must be agreed to) by existing cultural models, practices, and ways of thinking and being.

And so in this context, it is evident that the move towards ethical fortification is greatly benefited by the narrative articulation and construction of a 'community of concern' (Madigan and Epston, 1995, p. 257) or 'club of life' whose membership can be revised in accordance with the person's purposes (White, 1997, p. 22). Madigan (2007) describes such a community as one made up 'of re-membering and loving others who (hold) the stories of the client' (p. 186). This club can be seen as a counterpart to the community of subjection I discussed in earlier chapters. Specifically, while the community of subjection refers to those in the person's life (whose number may include the person himself or herself) who often unwittingly support his or her problem-saturated identity and hold him or her to it, the club of life refers to those (again, including the person himself or herself) who support preferred developments and are in some way able to participate with the person in the performance of his or her ethically informed stance. In my view, the primary purpose of the supportive community is to produce an ensemble of socially aligned activities which serves to support the person's location in a particular, preferred set of subject positions. As such, we need not be prescriptive about its membership. It can include persons, animals, plants, living or deceased, or groups of individuals, such as teams, nations, or other social categories. Sometimes one can hold on to one's own ethical subjectivity through identification with a particular group (e.g., citizens, animal rights activists, cancer survivors), supported by its juxtaposition against some perceived other (e.g., terrorists, pharmaceutical companies, cancer). My point is only that we need not limit our thought about communities (of subjection or concern) to specific, or even human, individuals.

And just as communities of subjection learn or evolve over time to respond in more nuanced and often more effective ways to render us subject to their requirements (as we saw in Chapter 3), so communities of concern can evolve to respond, together with us and sometimes for us, in increasingly sophisticated and creative ways to those forces which threaten to dislodge us from our preferred positions and ethical stances. To take a simple example, Carl's father's recollection of aspects of Carl's life that he himself could not remember, helped lend nuance to Carl's appreciation of the different ways he could speak up or oppose the abuse of power. Specifically, his father's recollection of Carl's response to the television drama depiction of a man's verbal assault on a woman led to an interesting discussion between us, in which we realized that standing up to bullying included, for Carl, a previously unarticulated opposition to gender-based violence and other forms of inequality. Carl's community of support had, in this instance, effectively facilitated the evolution and expansion of the values he stood for into new and unexpected territories. Our friends, loved ones, and even others who we do not know, can help us perform our values in new ways, and to bring them into new domains of our lives. This means, significantly, that we are not fortified as *static* ethical subjects. Our ethical subjectivity should not become a new form of discursive imprisonment. Rather, we become strong subjects through our dynamic participation in the ethical fields that open up, in spontaneous, emergent fashion, as a consequence of our identifications with and enactments of those principled positions.

It is important to note that the distinction between communities of concern and communities of subjection is a discursive or narrative distinction, and as such we cannot assume anything so neat as mutually exclusive membership. We will recall that persons are always multi-storied and multiply constituted, which means that they might support and frustrate our different initiatives or forms of subjection in a complex, unpredictable mixture of ways. And so, of course, these two 'types' of communities will likely have overlapping membership. One community member might support the problem, or some aspect of the person's unwanted identity conclusions, while at other moments, or when speaking from other positions in the context of our inevitable multiplicity, that community member might assist the person in standing against these.

It is against the backdrop of such variable and complex recruitments that benefit may be found in a careful engagement with some community members in the therapeutic process itself, such as in definitional ceremonies (e.g., White, 2007). These club members – friends, family members, colleagues, etc. – are not given carte blanche in these discussions, because to do so would invite a complex mix of supports of and impediments to the values and principles that form part of the person's initiatives. A reconstituting community could not easily be formed under such conditions.

I recall a difficult situation many years ago, when I was one of five members of a reflecting team working with a family. Some team members noted some interesting developments in one particular family member's life. This was a 16-year-old girl, who appeared to have moved from hating her father in previous sessions to expressing tenderness towards him in this session. In the session, the therapist noted this tenderness, and her mother indicated that she was a very loving person 'underneath it all'. When it came time for our reflecting session, with the family listening and watching us through the mirror, many of us found ourselves drawn to this movement. But then one practitioner declared, in full view of the team and the family, that the young woman had a 'borderline personality' and that what we were witnessing was 'splitting behaviour'. Clearly, at a formal, theoretical level, we could not function as a supportive club because we were not contributing to the same form of reconstitution. On the one hand, some team members were opening up space – in line with the family's dialogue – for the young person's repositioning in some as yet undetermined way; perhaps as a loving daughter, or as someone who valued family and love. But on the other hand, she was also being positioned as a disturbed young woman who was split in two and destined to cause confusion in the family.

And so in definitional ceremonies, in which a community of persons is invited to witnesses and participate in the person's developments, White emphasizes that a significant amount of therapeutic work is required to promote clarity in their orientation to the conversation, such that what is elicited is a directed, even disciplined, form of support. For example, the direction taken includes an attempt to 'regrade' rather than 'judge and degrade' the person's life (White, 2007, p. 165), and to contribute to 'building a sense of solidarity with regard to the values and aspirations for life reflected in (the person's)...personal narratives' (White, 2007, p. 179). In other words, the recruited community is asked to orient to the person and his or her values in a particular way. White does not leave this to chance, and advocates very carefully 'repositioning' participants before they offer their reflections on the person's developments. Their participation is not free and open ended, but restricted to a specific series of questions, themes, or 'categories of inquiry' (p. 190), determined by the therapist, so that they 'disengage from their habitual ways of responding' to the person (p. 202 – for more on this practice, see White, 2007, Chapter 4).

So, in the terms of our discussion of the fortification of the ethical subject, we recognize that the expressions and activities of communities of concern, if they are to function effectively as supports of preferred developments and as aids against unwanted forces of constitution, must in some respects become aligned so as to contribute to the formation of an alternative power/knowledge system and a new set of inhabitable positions. And to the extent that this alignment is realized, even if only in a few key moments and around a few vital issues, it serves to powerfully supplement the ethical subject's strivings, and thereby to strengthen his or her principled position.

The careful setting-up required for definitional ceremonies is testament to the fact, already suggested by Deleuze (1988), that the maintenance and upkeep of a particular form of ethical subjectivity is a quite significant achievement. In the person's day-to-day life, people will respond in multiple ways, and not necessarily in line with the steps he or she is taking. It is in such circumstances that we might become concerned about the person being 'blown by the wind' of these various forces, putting him or her at risk of being recuperated by the initial constituting discourse and its problematic positions. But the ethically fortified subject, equipped with personal stories and a history thickened with references to his or her practice in the enactment of certain principles or values, and who is supported *in some way* by an identifiable community of actors, is able to buttress himself or herself against these winds, and to hold firm in the ethical forms he or she has adopted.

The intensification of social relations

What emerges is an image of the person as existing in a thoroughly antagonistic social situation. Discourse theorists Laclau and Mouffe (e.g., 2001) are perhaps most explicit about this, in their depiction of identity as given shape in the context of a social world constituted by battles between discourses competing for centredness. And of course, the work of Foucault persuasively shows the immanence of power in discourse and societal dynamics. This is not to say that people or communities have malevolent intentions, or that those deemed powerful control discourses at the expense of the weak or powerless. Rather, our commitment is to the view that we – all of us, regardless of social, economic, or political position – exist in a broad field of power dynamics from which escape into something like 'non-power' is ultimately impossible. It is in the context of *this environment* that the ethical subject is called into being. This is a subject with an inherent and embodied capacity for resistance, entailing a refusal to be fixed in one identity position for all time, and who is able to capitalize on this resistance through the more socialized and intentional utilization of discursive 'equipment' (e.g., socially available ideas, practices, beliefs) to cultivate a personal ethos. This allows the person to make meaning of his or her refusals, to construct commitments, and to thereby stand firm even when caught up in the raging storms of power. Ethics is the 'conscious practice of freedom', the deliberate form we give to our refusals of what is, and to our subversions of the constituted forms into which we have been made (Foucault, 1997d, p. 284). Raw, 'animal' refusal and excess can thus be narratively thickened, and nuanced into a socially usable, meaning-filled, and ethically informed stance.

And so we arrive at the fourth, and perhaps most vital feature of the ethical subject. This figure, like all of us, is always situated in power dynamics, but his or her principled position renders him or her an active participant in those dynamics. Instead of being pushed and pulled by power, the ethical subject has found a personally resonant, more or less anchored, but also socially relevant or recognizable position from which to resist certain forms of power, while moving with those directions of power that align with his or her intentions, commitments, values, and, perhaps, with the ethos or style of being that he or she has chosen to cultivate. In this sense, the ethical subject is capable of critical political participation (Gros, 2005), and engages in intensified social relations. By this, I do not mean that he or she is always up for a fight, or that he or she necessarily advocates for social justice, lobbies for change, or organizes marches to signal protest against rape or some other form of injustice (although, of course, such actions might flow from one's commitments). Instead, I am referring to politics with a small 'p' (see also White, 2004). This is a vision of the person as one who is able to engage intentionally and from a given stance with the local, micro politics of life.

By virtue of the fact that we are all simultaneously effects and vehicles of power, the ethical subject stands as both product and representative of a particular set of (culturally available and recognizable) values or commitments. This means not only that he or she is subject to them, but also that he or she is thereby equipped to invite others, in the manner of an interpellation, into his or her club of life, and to call others into intensified and personally meaningful social participation.

This recruiting capacity was evident in my work with Oscar (see Chapter 3), who had been assaulted by his ex-wife and came to see himself as a failure of a man. His recognition of the discursively prescribed subject position he had come to occupy led to a proliferation of resistances and initiatives. In terms of our current focus on ethical subjectivity, it is worth noting that in our discussions Oscar had come to the realization that his new partner's understanding of him – not as a failure but as 'a gentle, quiet soul who comes through when it counts' – reflected something that was important to him; and furthermore, it was something not determined by the hegemonic discourses of masculinity that had come to define his identity. As we discussed further, he told me that the problem with the world, as he saw it, was that very often people did not try to 'understand' other people. And so if he was one who 'comes through when it counts', it was because he tried to understand, rather than discount, those people whose actions confused him. So, understanding was identified as something he gave significant value to. To Oscar, understanding meant not judging, and not criticizing people, but trying to appreciate and consider what they were going through. He said, 'you can't tell just looking at someone what they're like, you can't just make up your mind if you don't understand what they've been through'. Interestingly, Oscar had made the decision to set up a self-led discussion group in a public hall for men who had experienced abuse. He effectively constructed a club, comprising a group of individuals who he felt might understand him, and in turn he wanted to try and understand what they had gone through and how they had dealt with it. I never met with these men, but it struck me that Oscar's resistance against his forms of subjection had not only equipped him to find other ways of thinking about and conducting himself, but also to recruit others who had been similarly positioned into rethinking their ways of being in the world. Effectively, guided by the value of understanding, Oscar initiated a particular club of life, inviting its members through mutual understanding to move away from the problem-saturated conclusions they (he expected) might have reached about themselves.

But the social intensifications associated with the assumption of an ethical subjectivity do not always result in such ambitious and potentially far-reaching initiatives. In Carl's situation, his adherence to the value of speaking truth to power meant that in certain social situations he would speak up instead of being silent. In Liam's work with Michael White (2007), his identification with fairness and salvaging life made possible an act of 'reaching out' to contact an old friend he had not seen for some time, but who had 'been through a lot' (p. 73). And Hollie, in conversation with Jill Freedman, declared that instead of keeping silent about her harassment and passively accepting that she could not have a raise in her job, she would 'make a point of doing something', 'cause trouble', and even file 'a harassment suit' (Freedman and Combs, 1996, p. 168). Each person's steps towards what we have been referring to as an ethical subjectivity – a subjectivity, that is, informed by some sense of right and wrong, by a sense of what is precious or valuable to the person, and a sense of a style or ethos of living – involves him or her in an intentionally focused and active engagement in the world, in a biased, directional, side-taking, and hence socially intensified way.

Oscar's understanding, Carl's standing up to bullying, Liam's salvaging of life, Hollie's heeding of her own voice: each stands as a fortified nexus, a meeting point, of preferences, ideas, stories, memories, values, relationships, and social practices, whose interwoven strands have the potential to give it a density and a resilience that helps fracture the grip that the forces of social constitution might otherwise have had. This nexus is the culmination, the coming to fruition, of a disciplined and active rather than a free and contemplative quest to locate oneself as an *individual* in a universe of social power relations. On the Nietzschean reading, according to Smith, the person exists as 'a nothing' and requires 'discipline' (Smith, p. 149) in order to become *something*: it requires discipline, focus, and intention to become one who can engage actively and agentively with power. The person's participation in a world infused with power dynamics is intensified insofar as his or her ethical stance speaks directly to power and functions as a resistance: that 'most intense point of a life, the point where its energy is concentrated, ... where it comes up against power, struggles with it, attempts to use its forces and to evade its traps' (Foucault, 2000a, p. 162). The ethical position is inevitably a socially intensified one.

Distinguishing between the ethical and the constituted subject

Finally, I wish to offer some thoughts on the distinction between the ethical and the constituted subject, given that each can involve some degree of ethical commitment as well as some degree of subjection. This distinction might be useful, not to 'diagnose' or categorize a particular individual as either constituted or ethical, but to help us avoid the traps of the former, and to think through our own therapeutic orientations to the people with whom we work. It might further help clarify our commitment to the nature of persons' active participation in the power dynamics of their lives.

We saw earlier that Foucault invoked the image of a passive figure, blown around by the winds of discourse, as a stark contrast against which to consider the ethical subject. But in some ways this contrast is misleading. The passive figure he describes is not quite the figure produced by the forces of social constitution, but is more reminiscent of Agamben's (1999) account of the 'Musselman' in Auschwitz; the Jewish detainee in a Nazi concentration camp who has lost the will to live, and who has become detached from all meaningful subject positions. I think a more useful contrast is with what we might consider the real other of the ethical subject: the constituted subject. I suggest that these two figures are not two opposites, existing on different poles of a continuum, ranging from, perhaps, obedient to agentive. It seems to me rather that *both* figures are in some measure docile, obedient, and, in a manner of speaking, agentive. We have seen that constituted figures, just like their ethical counterparts, will often fight very hard in defence of their ways of being and knowing. So the distinction between the two, theoretically speaking, is rather slippery. Veyne (2010) has discussed how an ethos or style of life that proves useful can under certain conditions evolve into a social expectation to which we must be obedient: ethos becomes subjection. For instance, a certain ethos (e.g., the protestant work ethic described by Max Weber – see Weber, Baehr, and Wells, 2002) might be widely valorized, become entrenched and expected in various social practices, linked up with religious or capitalist goals, and so on. It easily becomes a socially prescribed, rather than personal-ethical, way of being. Similarly, on the other hand, persons inevitably evolve a personal ethos out of their investments in particular forms of subjection. From where else could this ethos originate? The difference between the constituted and the ethical subject is not so easily found in one's support of or resistance against prevailing power relations and arrangements.

Nor do we find the difference in the *contents* of the principles or values to which the constituted or ethical subject is committed. We cannot say, a priori, that one's honesty, sense of fairness, or opposition to bullying, are not already products of the person's constitution as a subject. We have seen at the beginning of this chapter that constituted subjects are also constituted as moral, valuing subjects, who have become invested in certain ways of thinking and being. Nor can we disqualify the striving for self-improvement, the quest to become more 'manly', or a person's investment in a romantic life, as valid forms of ethical existence. The contents of one's commitments do not serve as reliable signals either of the person's cultivation of a personal ethos in the context of power, or of his or her subjection to power's requirements.

Nevertheless, as I see it there are three major ways in which the ethical subject can be conceptually distinguished from the constituted subject (remembering that we are always, to some extent, both), and that is in terms of their respective relationships to (1) the living, embodied human being who seeks both to accept and resist subjection (2) the other, and (3) life in general.

First, it seems to me that the embodied figure described in Chapter 5 – who seeks both subjection and freedom – is granted more space to realize both of these objectives when construed in terms of ethical self-formation than in terms of self-knowledge. In order to appreciate this, let us recall two of the primary Nietzschean assumptions I made about the human being, which, I have argued, underpins persons' subjectification. On the one hand, in order to live this being must believe in and attach unquestioning value to *something* (Nietzsche, 1968, p. 276), which then comes to ground its activities and identity – even though the *contents* of this believed something are not predetermined, a priori, in the absence of particular social, cultural, and historical circumstances. This requirement that we believe and value something is what makes us susceptible to the social forces of subjection, which in turn provide us with specific 'somethings' to believe in and value. And then on the other hand, I argued for the view, which some see lying implicit in

Foucault's own work, that this being must be allowed to perform its inherent multiplicity, and in the process occasionally overcome or overflow the something it believes in and has come to be. This is what makes negative resistance possible. These two assumptions may be thought of as conditions of life (which is how we sometimes find them described by Nietzsche and, perhaps more implicitly, by Foucault), and correspond, respectively, to the human being's orientation to subjection *and* freedom (or resistance).

The constituted and the ethical subject appear to engage with these hypothesized conditions of human life in very different ways. On the one hand, the constituted subject, who is oriented to the self-defining question 'Who am I?', reifies and personalizes the first of these conditions. Life's requirement that something should 'be held to be true' is reified by its conflation with its historically and culturally specific iteration: a search for *the* truth, and a subsequent declaration that this truth '*is* true' (Nietzsche, 1968, p. 276). And then, this truth requirement is personalized. That is, not only must we believe in the existence of absolute truth in general terms, but we must also believe in, and discover, the truth about *ourselves*. So a constituted subject is born, taking the form of an apparently stable, predictable, and knowable identity: this is the truth about oneself. Thus, the emphasis here is on the person as a subjection-affirming being who can be known in some truthful, finalized sense: 'I am this!' – a murderer, a failure of a man, incompetent, dependent, a loose woman. And while many of these identity conclusions are unwanted and distressing, they nevertheless satisfy the cultural requirement (as opposed to Nietzsche's requirement of *life*) that the constituted subject prioritize the truth about *itself*.

But these personalized truths amount to a curtailment of the second condition: the human being's freedom to perform its inherent multiplicity. In a sense, even the subject constituted in negative, unwanted ways is effectively persuaded to trade his or her freedom for truth; for the reassurances of belonging, certainty, and 'security' (Klossowski, 2005, p. 80), and for the promise of being held in the 'loving embrace' of discourse and power (Prozorov, 2007b, p. 62). For example, we saw in Michael White's work with Judy (see Chapter 4), who had been recruited into the culture of self-help and self-improvement, and its valorization of independence and competence, that these ideals promised her so much: a sense of accomplishment, the security of knowing who she should be, the security of knowing that she is just one of many in her culture on the self-improvement path, a sense, therefore, of belonging, as well as an assurance of a good and fulfilling life to come, just around the corner, with a little more effort...Her sense of failing to reach these goals does not detract from their 'loving embrace'. But these promises also obscure and curtail her freedom – to resist, and to move onto other life projects. In other words, in its valorization of a singular, imposed truth which shapes the contents of a person's identity, constituted subjectivity effectively closes down his or her dynamic multiplicity.

On the other hand, the notion of the ethical subject, who orients to the question 'how shall I conduct myself?', seems to grant the human being space to move between both of these conditions and thereby to honour their dynamic interrelationship. In contrast to the constituted subject, the ethical subject seeks not to become a certain *type* of person – his or her 'true self' – but to conduct his or her life in accordance with certain principles that exist in the broader culture. The problem Judy has is that her 'failure' to attain the self-improvement standards set for her leads her to conclude that she is, in herself, a 'failure': weak, dependent, incompetent. But the ethical position into which she moves through the therapeutic conversation – labelled an 'ethic of partnership' – refers not to a reified and personalized self-knowledge or identity, or some static, predetermined goal, but to an ongoing, intentional, and trans-formable practice of partnering with others. *Something* – in this case, partnership – can be believed in and given value, as Nietzsche says, but it need not reify or define the person who is doing the believing. Sim-ilarly, Carl's decision to speak up when it is difficult, even though it was initially associated with his quest to be 'true to himself', involves no fixed identity claims. In our conversation we do not pin down who this 'himself' is, but work instead with the value he places on speak-ing up and opposing abuses of power, and which have the potential to allow him to be more fully present and engaged in his life. Thus, with respect to the first condition (believing and valuing something), in the ethical subject we see a shift in emphasis: from believing in a truth about oneself, to believing in and valuing certain principles, which in turn allow one to avoid being pinned down as a certain kind of person.

And then, with respect to the condition of inherent multiplicity, we should note that the cultivation of a personal ethos is not considered a once-and-for-all attainment, but is based on living, contingent prin-ciples that must be adapted and diversified as life moves on. In other words, ethical subjectivity affords a degree of fluidity and multiplicity. This was evident in my work with Carl, whose commitment to 'tackling the bullying nonsense' spread in unpredictable ways into other areas of his life, inspiring him at a later point, for example, to declare his love for a particular woman. There is no fixed principle – not even his 'self' – that could have predicted that his stand against bullying would lead to a declaration of love, precisely because the practice of ethics involves an adaptability and dynamic responsiveness to life's unpredictable and contingent circumstances and contexts. Ethical subjectivity multiples rather than reduces practice possibilities.

And yet this is not a chaotic endeavour. There is an 'ethos' – a discipline – at work in both Judy's and Carl's lives: a sense of acting in line with what is important to them, even though the definition of that 'important thing' will vary, depending on what life presents.

In other words, the ethical subject is freer than the constituted subject by virtue of the fact that this person (1) is not tied to a particular identity and is not expected to ground himself or herself on some supposedly inner, essential truth, and (2) intentionally follows guiding principles which are found on the outside, in the contingent and changeable contexts of a life in progress. Thus, in terms of the two hypothesized conditions of the human animal, the ethical subject is defined neither by the strictures of discursive constitution, nor by the multiple, formless flows of his or her own embodied excess; neither sculpted into a docile puppet, nor dissolved into chaos. Its responsiveness to contingent life circumstances means that it must construct and reconstruct itself in an ongoing way, and therefore apply a flexible approach to its own discipline, which never amounts to a fixed identity. Ethical subjectivity permits an ongoing and dynamic flow, backwards and forwards, between the discipline of commitment and the creativity of overflowing multiplicity. It allows and facilitates a somewhat fluid and dynamic relationship between subjection and resistance, between the social and the individual, and between the singular and the multiple, without losing sight of either aspect. And it can do so because the person orients to the question of how he or she should live, rather than to the question of who he or she 'is'. If, to paraphrase Foucault, constitution imprisons the body and its conduct, then ethical subjectivity is a way of opening up, albeit in structured, disciplined, even discursively styled fashion, spaces for dynamic activity and self-reinvention. This, in my view, is the significance of Foucault's thought of shifting the question we use to orient to ourselves and our lives: from knowledge of the self to an ethics of the self.

The second distinction we can make between the constituted and ethical subject concerns the orientation to the other. As constituted subjects, we are compelled to act towards the other in terms of the truths we hold about ourselves and each other. For example (and as discussed extensively in Chapter 3), we frequently engage in normative judgements and other regulating and monitoring (though often well-meaning) practices to insure that a person is obedient to the truth of who he or she is, as we understand it. We greet the widow, determined to live again, who has decided to go out for a cup of coffee after a lonely year of grieving, with sympathy, with sad expressions, tilted heads, a warm tone of voice, and heartfelt hugs as we reassure her that she should not be afraid to cry. We inadvertently undermine her intentions – this is precisely not what she wants – by acting on the basis of what we consider to be the truth about her: she is a sad, lonely person, who is despairing and grieving. And so we hold her to it.

But the ethical subject – whose intentionality and deliberate identi-fication with particular principles assists him or her to recognize that these principles are not truths but practical and stylistic guidelines – displays an 'openness to the other' (Falzon, 1998, p. 12). We allow the other to move, and to not be who we think they should be. This open-ness consists in an honouring of the other's needs for both a soft, flexible form of subjection – or way of being known – as well as the freedom to exceed that position and move into other ways of being and knowing. Essentially, this entails a willingness to respect the other's freedom to invent and reinvent himself or herself, and to have the freedom to be something other than we would like him or her to be, rather than tie him or her to some truth about who he or she should be. It entails a respect of the other's participation in society's games of power in ways that might or might not line up with our own ethical prefer-ences, or with our own sense of what is 'right' or 'wrong'. This is the Foucauldian ethics Falzon (1998) describes, and it coheres with a perfor-mative respect for the other as one who is constituted in a dynamic and never-ending relationship between subjection on the one hand, and multiplicity, resistance, and overflowing on the other. It does not involve 'knowing' the other, which is to constrain him or her in par-ticular forms of subjection, and to simultaneously deny him or her the freedom to expand into his or her inherent multiplicity and to partici-pate in societal games of power in his or her own way. The ethical subject has an 'openness to the other', through which others are seen, in turn, as ethical rather than constituted subjects.

But this reluctance to impose a final understanding on the other, and to respect his or her choices, values, and ethics, is not to say that 'any-thing goes', and that we should support all causes and actions. We must remember that we are always within fields of power, and in order to retain their dynamic nature and to protect against hegemonization, we too must somewhere, somehow, take sides. What do we do about sexist, homophobic, or racist practices? Can these stand as legitimate ways of practising ethical subjectivity? While they may involve intentional commitments, such practices tend to reify others, fix them to certain identities, and thereby systematically close down opportunities for them to experience their own freedom. Thus, Thiele (1990), citing the Ku Klux Klan as an example, argues that styles of being that exclude others from creative self-invention and active participation in the power dynamics of their lives can be considered 'condemnable' (p. 922).

It seems to me that the styles of being associated with such practices are problematic, from a Foucauldian perspective, not precisely because of their *contents*, but because of their *effects*. In light of this, if we consider our commitment to a social space which opens up rather than closes down positional and ethical possibilities – this is, perhaps, the primary 'side' that the narrative practitioner takes – we might be in a position to establish limits regarding what kinds of ethical subjectivity we would find tolerable. While the issue is not always so clear-cut, I have found Falzon's notion of a 'dialogue of forces' (1998, p. 43) to be helpful. This suggests we should resist any practice that impedes persons' capacities to participate in this dialogue – which must never be allowed to become fully a one-way monologue or hegemony of forces – and thereby to change aspects of their lives. We can advocate resistance against self-styled practices that preclude others' abilities to meaningfully resist the forms imposed on them, and which hold persons in deadening, degrading, and finalized positions.

The third distinction I wish to make is already implicit in the above discussion. While the subject of knowledge – the constituted subject – is a figure or being ('I am ... '), the ethical subject must be a figure of becoming ('I am striving to ... '). It is in this context that we can understand the claim of Nietzsche's Zarathustra: 'I am *that which must always overcome itself* ... Whatever I create and however much I love it – soon I must oppose it and my love' (Nietzsche, 2006, pp. 89–90, emphasis in original). The meaning of this is well articulated by Reginster (2007), who says that for Nietzsche the living organism does not so much seek to *'achieve'* as it seeks to be *'achieving'*. The reduction of ethos ('this is how I am living my life') to logos ('this is who I am') – and one might frequently be enticed by practices and communities of power/knowledge to effect just such a conversion, as they seek to tell us who we are, or require that we tell them – is, on this view, a movement from dynamism to stasis; in Reginster's terms, from a sense of achieving to a sense of having achieved. A person's sense of having finally attained a particular form of ethical subjectivity, as if it were now forever anchored in his or her being, risks eventually frustrating his or her inherent multiplicity and impulse towards dynamism, and hence, I have proposed, may evoke disequilibrating manoeuvres. Even the most prized subject positions are subject to disruption as the living being overflows them. But the consequent opening up of new forms of ethical living still requires intentional work. The ethical being is always in a state of becoming. In order to avoid being reduced to a stultified, constituted subject, the ethical subject must perform the ongoing destruction and recreation of his or her ways of being.

One implication of this is that we should take care in our practices not to reduce ethos to logos, personal ethics to self-knowledge. This is how I make sense of the narrative practitioner's wariness of internal state forms of understanding, which threaten to convert an ethical style into a marker of who the person 'is', rather than considering it a dynamic, living, intentional activity, oriented to the question of how one is trying in an ongoing way to live one's life. Indeed, in my view, narrative practice strives to orient to the person not as someone who 'is' this or that, but as someone who is never concluded, never finalized, but always becoming.

I wonder if the notion of the ethical subject, which opens up a view of the person as always becoming, as always able to move between subjection and resistance while never denying the significance of either, might serve as a kind of culmination of narrative practice. It seems to me that it gives us, as practitioners, an image of what we have always suspected, indeed, what we have always counted on: that the person is a dynamic, always unfinalized being, who searches for the most promising forms of subjection that society says he or she is entitled to, but who never *quite* fits into the categories and stories he or she finds. Indeed, we recognize that the questions that constitute our lives – 'Who are you?' and 'Who am I?' – lead to an imprisonment of the person's inherent multiplicity, and so we work with him or her to find new territories of life in which at least some of this multiplicity might be given room to breathe. We strive to honour this person's freedom, which is not a radical freedom to be anything, or even to be himself or herself, but the freedom to say 'no', to journey without having to choose a final destination, to be always becoming. The freedom, too, to refuse the question society demands he or she answer, and to ask a different one.

Conclusion: Who is the person in narrative therapy?

The death of man, heralded by Foucault, does not require the erasure of the agentive human individual, only of the *essential* being, the human who can be known and understood as one thing, once and for all time. The constituted subject, who obediently mirrors himself or herself on this essentialized image, seeks the elusive inner truth of itself; that once-and-for-all thing that it supposes it is. But the notion of the ethical subject, through its honouring of the human being's inherent multiplicity, highlights the impossibility of this task, and represents a recognition of the person's unfinalizable nature; of his or her virtually endless capacity to resist enclosure within essentializing systems of knowledge, to disrupt and reveal the incompleteness of socially constituted identity forms, and thus to exceed the limits of the 'self' he or she has come to be.

On this account, ethical subjectivity is a feature of life that human beings are already oriented to. Valuing – which the ethical subject orients to in a very particular way – is essential to life itself, as Nietzsche has told us. But it is society which guides us on which values to uphold. Foucault hints that we might have oriented to a value that has set us off on problem-saturated paths; we have been asking and trying to answer the wrong question. Specifically, Foucault, following Nietzsche, showed that historical and cultural forces have pressed us to value *knowledge*, and in particular *self-knowledge*, above all else. And so we obediently try to find ourselves in that place – of knowledge – to provide the true answer to the question, 'Who am I?' Our greatest value, we have been led to believe, lies in answer to that question. To my mind, one of Foucault's most astounding achievements was to show that it is this that makes us especially vulnerable to particular forms of subjection, through which we come to form conclusions about who we are. But these conclusions, as White has noted, are inevitably one-dimensional, single-voiced, and take on normative, governing qualities: some conclusions – some identities – are deemed better than others. And for many, these conclusions are limiting and oppressive. They might promote a sense of oneself as inferior, as hopelessly stuck with a devalued identity, and as lacking in any sense of personal agency.

So, significantly, Foucault calls not for an intensified drive to attain the most sought-after identities, but for a refusal of who we have become, and even a refusal of the restrictive question society demands we answer; an answer to which we are then held. The power game, after all, is rigged; and so we need to reject it and find another way. And, for me, this is where the narrative therapeutic project finds its purpose, its *raison d'être*. We aim to support people in their refusals of who they have been made into, not so that they can become more successful in society's normative games, but so that they can move, experientially, into a different kind of game – a game that privileges ethos rather than logos. The refusal of what one has become requires resistance, but, as I have argued, it is always already there. We do not have to persuade or educate the person on the question of what should be resisted. Resistance, that capacity to signal the presence of a stifling constitution, is already there: in our bodies, our actions, and our speech. It is everywhere, if we can just learn how to see it. It is already part of who we are, emerging as the response of our inherent multiplicity to the reductive effects of discourse and power. On this point, I have taken up a post-structural Nietzschean position: I see this multiplicity not as a socialized or culturally prescribed part of the human being, but, precisely, as an *essential* part of our make-up. It is this that allows us to distance ourselves from some values, and to find ourselves in a search for others – to move. And so we can imagine moving from the valorization of a reified self-knowledge to the privileging of a responsive and contingent personal ethos, informed by ethics, values, principles, and commitments.

I have found this vision of the human being as multiple and unfinalizable to be very useful in my therapeutic practice, as it has alerted me to the multiple and complex ways in which people, in their words, and sometimes in their very body movements, overflow or say 'no!' to the forms that have been imposed on them. I am struck by the diversity and raw energy of the embodied figure sitting in front of me. The practitioner does not narratively construct this multiplicity, or the bristling, living resistance it produces, but *recognizes* it, and then moves to thicken some of its strands into story form, and into values, ethics, principles, and commitments, through various re-storying, re-constituting technologies.

Such narrative technologies provide a kind of directionality in therapeutic conversations, nudging participants away from normalizing, constitutive, identify-fixing knowledges and practices, and towards the thickening of preferred ethical subjectivities and identities. After all, when we are governed by the question, 'Who am I?', we frequently find that there are few different places to move to. We could become better, faster, stronger, more manly, more beautiful; anything to move us up on the normative distribution curve. But through the articulation and exploration of one's ethical preferences, via the question, 'How should I live my life?', narrative practices seek to open up new vistas, which are not bound by the forms and choices foisted upon us. This allows the multiple, resisting figure, itself a nothing-in-particular, to be the becoming-something that it is; something more fluid, not quite so finalized as the being it was made into.

The narrative practitioner recognizes that the person is a moving, achieving, becoming-something. We recognize, and we seek to connect with, the person's endless capacity to make room for his or her own dynamism, life, and creative reinvention. This is something we can trust about the human being.

Glossary of Terms: Five Narrative Therapeutic Practices

Definitional ceremonies and outsider witnessing – Often in narrative practice significant others are invited in to stand as 'outsider witnesses' to the person's preferred developments. In response to the person's 'telling' of these developments, the witnesses are invited, in a 're-telling' process, to reflect on what struck a chord for them, and to connect resonant themes with their own lives. The therapist carefully structures this witnessing as a kind of ceremony, in which talk is directed towards supporting the person's agentive stories, values, behaviours, and experiences. The ceremony can facilitate the emergence of new ideas and themes for further re-authoring and re-membering conversations, but its primary purpose is to begin a process of thickening and grounding the person's preferred ways of being in communal life and spaces (for further reading, see White, 2007, Chapter 4).

Externalization – Externalization is based on the idea that personal problems are the product of the internalization of the prescriptions and expectations of external discourse and power dynamics (although the term 'internalization' might be contentious in that Foucault tended to speak of social processes as inscribed 'on' the body, rather than internalized 'into' it). It refers to the conversational practice of separating the person from the problem, which is thereby externalized. In practice, this involves speaking about the problem as external to the person, and as exerting some kind of influence on him or her (e.g., the claim 'I am anorexic' might lead the therapist to ask questions such as: 'How does anorexia persuade you to treat your body?'). In the process, the problem and its specifications are delinked from the person's sense of self. The space that opens up between person and problem gives the person room to reconsider his or her relationship to the problem, and to reflect on his or her identity and life experience separately from the 'problem-saturated stories' promoted by the internalized discourse (see White, 2007, Chapter 1, and White and Epston, 1990, Chapter 2).

Re-authoring – This conversational practice involves the development of a personal history of those behaviours, thoughts, interactions, or other experiences which run counter to, or seem out of phase with, problem-saturated stories and the non-preferred thoughts, behaviours, and experiences they sponsor. The therapist asks questions that move back and forth between the 'landscape of action' (actual historical events and happenings in the person's life) and the 'landscape of identity' (what these events suggest about the person's identity, sense of agency, ethics, values, and commitments), in an attempt to narratively thicken, and to foster a sense of historical depth and personal congruence in relation to preferred personal developments (see White, 2007, Chapter 2).

Re-membering – The stories of preferred developments can be thickened by linking them up with others in the person's life. This may involve conversations about who should be told about an important personal realization, who might have already noticed it, who might support it, and in what ways. It also may involve discussing the mutual influences between the person and these others, so that an appreciation is gained not just of the others' support, but of the person's contributions to these others' lives. This bidirectional influence is important to articulate, as it helps promote a sense of mutual personal agency and of a mutually supportive community. The term 're-membering' is used because the person is seen as becoming a 'member' of an enabling community, which may have been forgotten or not fully recognized (see White, 2007, Chapter 3).

Unique outcomes – Narrative therapists assume that there will always be times in the person's life in which he or she subverts or resists the problem and its supporting narratives. When the person sees value in these out-of-phase behaviours or experiences, they may be referred to as unique outcomes. These outcomes, which are often initially slight and barely noticed, then become the subject of numerous other narrative practices. For example, they may emerge out of externalizing conversations, and then be developed and narratively thickened in re-authoring, re-membering, and outsider-witnessing dialogues (see White, 2007, Chapter 5).

References

Agamben, G. (1999). *Remnants of Auschwitz: The Witness and the Archive* (trans. D. Heller-Raozen). New York: Zone Books.

Allen, A. (2000). 'The anti-subjective hypothesis: Michel Foucault and the death of the subject.' *The Philosophical Forum* 31(2), 113–130.

Althusser, L. (1971/2008). 'Ideology and ideological state apparatuses'. In L. Althusser, *On Ideology* (pp. 1–60). London: Verso.

Anderson, H. and Goolishian, H. (1990). 'Beyond cybernetics: comments on Atkinson and Heath's "Further thoughts on second order family therapy"'. *Family Process*, 29, 157–163.

Bakhtin, M. (1984). *Problems of Dostoevsky's Poetics*. London: University of Minnesota Press.

Bamberg, M. (2004). ' "We are young, responsible, and male": Form and function of "slut-bashing" in the identity construction in 15-year-old males'. *Human Development* 47, 331–352.

Bennett, J. (2005). 'The agency of assemblages and the North American blackout'. *Public Culture* 17(3), 445–465.

Bergeret, J. (2002). 'Homosexuality or homoeroticism? "Narcissistic eroticism"'. *International Journal of Psychoanalysis* 83, 351–362.

Besley, A. C. (2002). 'Foucault and the turn to narrative therapy'. *British Journal of Guidance & Counselling* 30, 125–143.

Bevir, M. (1999). 'Foucault and critique: deploying agency against autonomy'. *Political Theory*, 27, 65–84.

Bhaskar, R. (2008). *A Realist Theory of Science*. New York: Routledge.

Bird, J. (2004). *Talk that Sings: Therapy in a New Linguistic Key*. Auckland: Edge Press.

Bohart, A. C. and Greenberg, L. S. (1997). 'Empathy: Where are we and we do we go from here?' In A. C. Bohart and L. S. Greenberg (eds), *Empathy Reconsidered: New Directions in Psychotherapy* (pp. 419–450). Washington: American Psychological Association.

Borch-Jacobsen, M. (1988). *The Freudian Subject*. Stanford: Stanford University Press.

Burnette, M. (1995). 'Secrets: Essentialism in narrative therapy'. *Journal of Child and Youth Care* 10, 1–12.

Burr, V. (1995). *An Introduction to Social Constructionism*. London: Routledge.

Butler, J. (1989). 'Foucault and the paradox of bodily inscriptions'. *The Journal of Philosophy* 86(11), 601–607.

Butler, J. (1997). *The Psychic Life of Power: Theories of Subjection*. Stanford: Stanford University Press.

Callender, J. S. (1998). 'Ethics and aims in psychotherapy: A contribution from Kant'. *Journal of Medical Ethics*, 24, 274–278.

Carey, M. and Russel, S. (2003). 'Re-authoring: Some answers to commonly asked questions'. *International Journal of Narrative Therapy & Community Work* 3, 60–71.

Carey, M., Walther, S., and Russell, S. (2009). 'The absent but implicit: A map to support therapeutic enquiry'. *Family Process* 48(3), 319–331.

Chernin, K. (1981). *The Obsession: Reflections on the Tyranny of Slenderness.* New York: Harper and Row.

Chiang, S. Y. (2010). ' "Well, I'm a lot of things, but I'm sure not a bigot": Positive self-presentation in confrontational talk on racism'. *Discourse & Society* 21(3), 273–294.

Conway, D. W. (1999). 'Pas de deux: Habermas and Foucault in genealogical communication'. In S. Ashenden and D. Owens (eds), *Habermas contra Foucault* (pp. 60–89). London: Sage.

Cushman, P. (1995). *Constructing the Self, Constructing America.* New York: Perseus Publishing.

Deleuze, G. (1988). *Foucault* (trans. S. Hand). London: Continuum.

Deleuze, G. (1990). *Negotiations* (trans. M. Joughin). New York: Columbia University Press.

Deleuze, G. (2006). *Nietzsche and Philosophy.* New York: Continuum.

Dreyfus, H. L. and Rabinow, P. (1982). *Michel Foucault: Beyond Structuralism and Hermeneutics* (2nd edn). Chicago: University of Chicago Press.

Durrheim, K. (1997). 'Cognition and ideology: A rhetorical approach to critical theory'. *Theory & Psychology* 7, 747–768.

Duvall, J. and Beres, L. (2011). *Innovations in Narrative Therapy: Connecting Practice, Training, and Research.* New York: W. W. Norton & Co.

Eagleton, T. (1991). *Ideology: An Introduction.* London: Verso.

Engels, F. (1893). 'Letter to Mehring'. www.marxists.org/archive/mehring/1893/histmat/app.htm. Retrieved 7 May 2013.

Epston, D. (1993). 'Internalizing discourses versus externalizing discourses'. In S. Gilligan (ed.), *Therapeutic Conversations* (pp. 161–180). New York: W. W. Norton & Co.

Falk, P. (1985). 'Corporeality and its fates in history'. *Acta Sociologica* 28(2), 115–136.

Falzon, C. (1993). 'Foucault's human being'. *Thesis Eleven* 34, 1–16.

Falzon, C. (1998). *Foucault and Social Dialogue.* New York: Routledge.

Fish, V. (1999). 'Clementis's hat: Foucault and the politics of psychotherapy'. In I. Parker (ed.), *Deconstructing Psychotherapy* (pp. 54–70). London: Sage.

Florence, M. (1998). 'Foucault'. In J. D. Faubion (ed.), *Michel Foucault: Aesthetics, Method, and Epistemology* (pp. 459–463). London: Penguin.

Foucault, M. (1966). *The Order of Things.* New York: Routledge.

Foucault, M. (1972). *The Archaeology of Knowledge.* London: Tavistock.

Foucault, M. (1977). *Discipline and Punish.* London: Penguin Books.

Foucault, M. (1979). 'Power and norm: Notes'. In M. Morris and P. Patton (eds), *Michel Foucault: Power, Truth, Strategy* (pp. 59–66). Sydney: Feral Publications.

Foucault, M. (1980a). *Power/Knowledge: Selected Interviews and other Writings 1972–1977.* (Ed. C. Gordon). New York: Harvester Wheatsheaf.

Foucault, M. (1980b). 'Prison talk'. In C. Gordon (ed.), *Power/Knowledge: Selected Interviews and other Writings 1972–1977* (pp. 37–54). New York: Harvester Wheatsheaf.

Foucault, M. (1980c). 'Two lectures'. In C. Gordon (ed.), *Power/Knowledge: Selected Interviews and other Writings 1972–1977* (pp. 78–108). New York: Harvester Wheatsheaf.

Foucault, M. (1980d). 'The eye of power'. In C. Gordon (ed.), *Power/Knowledge: Selected Interviews and other Writings 1972–1977* (pp. 146–165). New York: Harvester Wheatsheaf.

Foucault, M. (1982). 'The subject and power'. In H. Dreyfus and P. Rabinow (eds), *Michel Foucault: Beyond Structuralism and Hermeneutics* (pp. 208–226). Brighton: The Harvester Press.

Foucault, M. (1983). 'Preface'. In G. Deleuze and F. Guattari (eds), *Anti-Oedipus: Capitalism and Schizophrenia* (trans. R. Hurley, M. Seem, and H. R. Lane) (pp. xi–xiv). Minneapolis: University of Minnesota Press.

Foucault, M. (1984). 'What is an author?' In P. Rabinow (ed.), *The Foucault Reader: An Introduction to Foucault's Thought* (pp. 101–120). New York: Penguin.

Foucault, M. (1988a). 'An aesthetics of existence'. In L. D. Kritzman (ed.), *Michel Foucault: Politics, Philosophy, Culture: Interviews and other Writings: 1977–1984* (pp. 47–56). New York: Routledge.

Foucault, M. (1988b). 'Power and sex'. In L. D. Kritzman (ed.), *Michel Foucault: Politics, Philosophy, Culture: Interviews and other Writings: 1977–1984* (pp. 110–124). New York: Routledge.

Foucault, M. (1990a). *The History of Sexuality, Volume 1: An Introduction.* London: Penguin.

Foucault, M. (1990b). *The History of Sexuality, Volume 3: The Care of the Self.* London: Penguin.

Foucault, M. (1992). *The Use of Pleasure: The History of Sexuality* (Vol. 2). Harmondsworth: Penguin.

Foucault, M. (1997a). 'What is critique?' In S. Lotringer and L. Hochroth (eds), *The Politics of Truth* (trans. L. Hochroth) (pp. 23–82). New York: Semiotext.

Foucault, M. (1997b). 'Sex, power and the politics of identity'. In P. Rabinow (ed.), *Michel Foucault: Ethics, Subjectivity and Truth* (pp. 163–173). New York: New Press.

Foucault, M. (1997c). 'On the genealogy of ethics: An overview of work in progress'. In P. Rabinow (ed.), *Michel Foucault: Ethics: Subjectivity and Truth, Volume 1* (pp. 253–280). New York: The New Press.

Foucault, M. (1997d). 'The ethics of the concern for self as a practice of freedom'. In P. Rabinow (ed.), *Michel Foucault: Ethics, Subjectivity and Truth* (pp. 281–302). New York: New Press.

Foucault, M. (1997e). 'What is Enlightenment?' In P. Rabinow (ed.), *Michel Foucault: Ethics, Subjectivity and Truth* (pp. 303–320). New York: New Press.

Foucault, M. (1998a). 'On the archaeology of the sciences'. In J. D. Faubion (ed.), *Michel Foucault: Aesthetics, Method, and Epistemology* (pp. 297–333). London: Penguin.

Foucault, M. (1998b). 'Structuralism and post-structuralism'. In J. D. Faubion (ed.), *Michel Foucault: Aesthetics, Method, and Epistemology* (pp. 433–458). London: Penguin.

Foucault, M. (2000a). 'Lives of infamous men'. In J. D. Faubion (ed.), *Michael Foucault: Power: The Essential Works, Volume 3* (pp. 157–175). New York, NY: Penguin.

Foucault, M. (2000b). 'Questions of method'. In J. D. Faubion (ed.), *Michel Foucault: Power: The Essential Works, Volume 3* (pp. 223–238). New York, NY: Penguin.

Foucault, M. (2000c). 'For an ethic of discomfort'. In J. Faubion (Ed.). *Michel Foucault: Power: The Essential Works, Volume 3* (pp. 443–448). New York: New York Press.

Foucault, M. (2001). *The Hermeneutics of the Subject: Lectures at the College de France 1981–1982.* Basingstoke: Palgrave Macmillan.

Frances, A. (2010). 'Opening Pandora's box: The 19 worst suggestions for DSM5'. *Psychiatric Times.* http://intraspec.ca/FrancesA_PsychiatricTimes110210.pdf. Retrieved 1 March 2013.

Fraser, N. (1989). *Unruly Practices: Power, Discourse and Gender in Contemporary Social Theory.* Cambridge: Polity Press.

Freedman, J. and Combs, G. (1996). *Narrative Therapy: The Social Construction of Preferred Realities.* New York: W. W. Norton & Co.

Freud, S. (1963). 'Constructions in analysis'. In J. Strachey (ed. and trans.), *The Standard Edition of the Complete Psychological Works of Sigmund Freud* (pp. 255–269). London: Hogarth.

Freud, S. (1900). 'The interpretation of dreams'. In J. Strachey (ed.), *The Standard Edition of the Complete Works of Sigmund Freud* (Volume 4, pp. ix–627). London: The Hogarth Press and the Institute of Psycho-analysis.

Geertz, C. (1979). 'From the native's point of view: On the nature of anthropological understanding'. In P. Rabinow and W. M. Sullivan (eds), *Interpretive Social Science* (pp. 225–241). Berkeley: University of California Press.

Gergen, K. (1999). *An Invitation to Social Construction.* London: Sage.

Gordon, N. (1999). 'Foucault's subject: An ontological reading'. *Polity,* 31, 395–414.

Gros, F. (2005). 'Le souci de soi chez Michel Foucault: A review of the hermeneutics of the subject: Lectures at the College de France 1981–1982'. *Philosophy & Social Criticism* 31(5–6), 697–708.

Guignon, C. B. (1993). 'Authenticity, moral values, and psychotherapy'. In C. B. Guignon (ed.), *The Cambridge Companion to Heidegger* (pp. 215–239). Cambridge: Cambridge University Press.

Guilfoyle, M. (2009). 'Theorizing relational possibilities in narrative therapy'. *Journal of Systemic Therapies* 28(2), 19–33.

Guilfoyle, M. (2011). 'The ethical subject in poststructural therapy'. *Journal of Systemic Therapies* 30(4), 1–15.

Gutting, G. (1994). 'Introduction: Michel Foucault: A user's manual'. In G. Gutting (ed.), *The Cambridge Companion to Foucault* (pp. 1–27). Cambridge: Cambridge University Press.

Habermas, J. (1987). *Knowledge and Human Interests* (trans. J. J. Shapiro). Cambridge: Polity Press.

Habermas, J. (1990). *The Philosophical Discourse of Modernity* (trans. F. G. Lawrence). Cambridge: MIT Press.

Habermas, J. (1993). *Justification and Application: Remarks on Discourse Ethics* (trans. C. Cronin). Cambridge: MIT Press.

Hall, S. (1985). 'Signification, representation, ideology: Althusser and the post-structuralist debates'. *Critical Studies in Mass Communication,* 2(2), 99–114.

Hall, S. (2000). 'Who needs "identity"?' In P. du Gay, L. Evans, and P. Redman (eds), *Identity: A Reader* (pp. 15–30). London: Sage.

Hare-Mustin, R. T. (1994). 'Discourses in the mirrored room: A postmodern analysis of therapy'. *Family Process,* 33(1), 19–35.

Haugh, S. (2008). 'A person-centred perspective'. In S. Haugh and S. Paul (eds), *The Therapeutic Relationship: Perspectives and Themes* (pp. 36–50). Ross-on-Wye: PCCS Books.

Heidegger, M. (1987). *Nietzsche: Volume III: The Will to Power as Knowledge and as Metaphysics* (trans. D. F. Krell). New York: Harper.

Heller, K. J. (1996). 'Power, subjectification and resistance in Foucault'. *SubStance* 25(1), 78–110.

Hill, N. (2013). *Think and Grow Rich*. New York: Tribeca Books.

Hoy, D. C. (2004). *Critical Resistance: From Poststructuralism to Post-Critique*. London: MIT Press.

Huijer, M. (1999). 'The aesthetics of existence in the work of Michel Foucault'. *Philosophy & Social Criticism* 25(2), 61–85.

Ingleby, D. (1985). 'Professionals as socialisers: The "psy complex"'. *Research in Law, Deviance, and Social Control* 7, 79–109.

Kendall, G. and Wickham, G. (1999). *Using Foucault's Methods*. London: Sage.

King, M. (2009). 'Clarifying the Foucault–Habermas debate: Morality, ethics, and "normative foundations"'. *Philosophy & Social Criticism* 35(3), 287–314.

Kirby, V. (1991). 'Corporeal habits: Addressing essentialism differently'. *Hypatia* 6(3), 4–24.

Kitzinger, C. and Perkins, R. (1993). *Changing our minds: Lesbian Feminism and Psychology*. New York: New York University Press.

Klossowski, P. (2005). *Nietzsche and the Vicious Circle*. London: Continuum.

Krause, S. R. (2008). *Civil Passions: Moral Sentiment and Democratic Deliberation*. New Jersey: Princeton University Press.

Laclau, E. and Mouffe, C. (2001). *Hegemony and Socialist Strategy: Towards a Radical Democratic Politics* (2nd edn). New York: Verso.

Lee, C. (2004). 'Agency and purpose in narrative therapy: Questioning the postmodern rejection of metanarrative'. *Journal of Psychology and Theology* 32(3), 221–231.

Lingis, A. (1977). 'The will to power'. In D. B. Allison (ed.), *The New Nietzsche* (pp. 37–63). New York: Dell.

Little, G. L. and Robinson, K. D. (1990). 'Reducing recidivism by changing how inmates think: The systematic approach of moral reconation therapy'. *American Jails*, 4(3), 12–16.

Lock, A., Epston, D., Maisel, R., and de Faria, N. (2005). 'Resisting anorexia/bulimia: Foucauldian perspectives in narrative therapy'. *British Journal of Guidance & Counselling* 33(3), 315–332.

Madigan, S. (2003). 'Injurious speech: Counter-viewing eight conversational habits of highly effective problems'. *International Journal of Narrative Therapy and Community Work* 2, 12–19.

Madigan, S. (2007). 'Anticipating hope within written and naming domains of despair'. In Flaskas, C., McCarthy, I. and Sheehan, J. (eds), *Hope and Despair in Narrative and Family Therapy: Adversity, Forgiveness and Reconciliation* (pp. 174–197). Hove: Brunner-Routledge.

Madigan, S. (2010). *Counter-viewing Questions*. Paper presented at the TC9 Narrative Therapy Conference, Vancouver, BC, Canada.

Madigan, S. (2011). *Narrative Therapy*. Washington: American Psychological Association.

Madigan, S. and Epston, D. (1995). 'From spy-chiatric gaze to communities of concern: From professional monologue to dialogue'. In S. Friedman (ed.), *The Reflecting Team in Action* (pp. 257–277). New York: Guilford Publications.

Malafouris, L. (2008). 'At the potter's wheel: An argument for material agency'. In L. Malafouris and C. Knappett (eds), *Material Agency: Toward a Non-Anthropocentric Approach* (pp. 19–36). New York: Springer.

Marx, C. and Engels, F. (1974). *The German Ideology*. London: : Lawrence and Wishart.

Miller, J. (2000). *The Passion of Michel Foucault*. Cambridge, MA: Harvard University Press.

Millon, T. (1999). *Personality-Guided Therapy*. New York: John Wiley & Sons.

Mills, S. (2003). *Michel Foucault*. London: Routledge.

Naffine, N. (1994). 'Possession: Erotic love in the law of rape'. *The Modern Law Review* 57, 10–37.

Nealon, J. T. (2008). *Foucault beyond Foucault: Power and its Intensifications since 1984*. Stanford: Stanford University Press.

Nietzsche, F. (1968). *The Will to Power* (trans. W. Kaufman and R. J. Hollingdale). New York, NY: Vintage.

Nietzsche, F. (2006). *Thus Spoke Zarathustra: A Book for All and None* (trans. A. Del Carro). Cambridge: Cambridge University Press.

Norris, C. (1994). ' "What is enlightenment?" Kant and Foucault'. In G. Gutting (ed.), *The Cambridge Companion to Foucault* (pp. 159–196). Cambridge: Cambridge University Press.

O'Leary, P. (1999). 'Liberation from self-blame: Working with men who have experienced childhood sexual abuse'. In D. Denborough and C. White (eds), *Extending Narrative Therapy* (pp. 159–190). Adelaide: Dulwich Centre Publications.

O'Leary, T. (2002). *Foucault and the Art of Ethics*. London: Continuum.

Orbach, S. (1978). *Fat Is a Feminist Issue*. New York: Paddington Press.

Parker, I. (2011). *Lacanian Psychoanalysis: Revolutions in Subjectivity*. New York: Routledge.

Patton, P. (1989). 'Taylor and Foucault on power and freedom'. *Political Studies*, 37, 260–276.

Potter, J. and Wetherell, M. (1987). *Discourse and Social Psychology: Beyond Attitudes and Behaviour*. London: Sage.

Prozorov, S. (2007a). *Foucault, Freedom and Sovereignty*. Aldershot, UK: Ashgate.

Prozorov, S. (2007b). 'The unrequited love of power: Biopolitical investment and the refusal of care'. *Foucault Studies* 4, 53–77.

Purvis, T. and Hunt, A. (1993). 'Discourse, ideology, discourse, ideology, discourse, ideology . . . ' *British Journal of Sociology* 44(3), 473–99.

Rabinow, P. (2003). *Anthropos Today: Reflections on Modern Equipment*. New Jersey: Princeton University Press.

Reginster, B. (2007). 'The will to power and the ethics of creativity'. In B. Leiter and N. Sinhababu (eds), *Nietzsche and Morality* (pp. 32–56). Oxford: Oxford University Press.

Rogers, C. R. and Sanford, R. (1989). 'Client-centred psychotherapy'. In H. I. Kaplan and B. J. Sadoclk (eds), *Comprehensive Textbook of Psychiatry, V* (pp. 1482–1501). Baltimore: Williams & Wilkins.

Rose, N. (1985). *The Psychological Complex: Psychology, Politics, and Society in England 1869–1939*. London: Routledge.

Rouse, J. (1994). 'Power/knowledge'. In G. Gutting (ed.), *The Cambridge Companion to Foucault* (pp. 95–122). Cambridge: Cambridge University Press.

Ryan, C. (2012). 'The subjectified and resisting corporeal body: a theoretical framework for examining subjugation and resistance'. *Limerick Papers in Politics and Public Administration*, 2, 1–25.

Said, E. (1986). 'Foucault and the imagination of power'. In D. C. Hoy (ed.), *Foucault: A Critical Reader* (pp. 149–155). London: Blackwell.

Sampson, E. (1993). *Celebrating the Other: A Dialogic Account of Human Nature*. San Francisco: Westview Press.

Scaturo, D. J. (2010). 'Insight oriented psychotherapy'. In I. B. Weiner and W. B. Craighead (eds), *The Corsini Encyclopaedia of Psychology Volume 2* (pp. 823–826). New Jersey: John Wiley & Sons.

Segal, L. (1986). *The Dream of Reality: Heinz von Foerster's Constructivism*. New York: Norton.

Shulman, D. (1996). 'Foreword II'. In S. Freedman and J. Combs (eds), *Narrative Therapy: The Social Construction of Preferred Realities* (pp. xii–xiii). New York: W. W. Norton & Co.

Skinner, B. F. (1953). *Science and Human Behaviour*. New York: Macmillan.

Smith, G. B. (1996). *Nietzsche, Heidegger, and the Road to Postmodernity*. Chicago: University of Chicago Press.

Stern, D. B. (1997). *Unformulated Experience: From Dissociation to Imagination in Psychoanalysis*. Mahwah, NJ: Analytic Press.

Taylor, C. (1986). 'Foucault on freedom and truth'. In D. Couzens Hoy (ed.), *Foucault: A Critical Reader*. Cambridge: Basil Blackwell.

Thiele, L. P. (1990). 'The agony of politics: The Nietzschean roots of Foucault's thought'. *American Political Science Review* 84(3), 907–925.

Torronen, J. (2001). 'The concept of subject position in empirical social research'. *Journal for the Theory of Social Behaviour* 31(3), 313–329.

Vanaerschot, G. (1990). 'The process of empathy: Holding and letting go'. In G. Lietaer, J. Rombauts, and R. Van Balen (eds), *Client Centred and Experiential Psychotherapy in the Nineties* (pp. 269–293). Leuven: Leuven University Press.

Veyne, P. (1993). 'The final Foucault and his ethics'. *Critical Inquiry* 20, 1–9.

Veyne, P. (1997). 'Foucault revolutionizes history'. In A. Davidson (ed.), *Foucault and his Interlocutors* (pp. 146–182). Chicago, IL: University of Chicago Press.

Veyne, P. (2010). *Foucault: His Thought, his Character*. Cambridge: Polity Press.

Wade, A. (1997). 'Small acts of living: Everyday resistance to violence and other forms of oppression'. *Contemporary Family Therapy* 19(1), 23–39.

Wartenburg, T. (1990). *The Forms of Power: From Domination to Transformation*. Philadelphia: Temple University Press.

Weber, M., Baehr, P. R., and Wells, G. C. (2002). *The Protestant Ethic and the 'Spirit' of Capitalism and other Writings*. New York: Penguin Classics.

Weberman, D. (2000). 'Are freedom and anti-humanism incompatible? The case of Foucault and Butler'. *Constellations* 7, 255–271.

Whitaker, C. (1982). 'Gatherings'. In J. R. Neill and D. P. Kniskern (eds), *From Psyche to System: The Evolving Therapy of Carl Whitaker* (pp. 365–375). New York: Guilford Press.

White, M. (1993). 'Commentary: The histories of the present'. In S. Gilligan and R. Price (eds), *Therapeutic Conversations* (pp. 121–135). New York: Norton.

White, M. (1997). *Narratives of Therapists' Lives*. Adelaide: Dulwich Centre Publications.

White, M. (2000). *Reflections on Narrative Practice: Essays and Interviews*. Adelaide: Dulwich Centre Publications.

White, M. (2003). 'Narrative practice and community assignments'. *International Journal of Narrative Therapy and Community Work* 2, 17–56.

White, M. (2004). *Narrative Practice and Exotic Lives: Resurrecting Diversity in Everyday Life*. Adelaide, South Australia: Dulwich Centre Publications.

White, M. (2006). 'Working with people who are suffering the consequences of multiple trauma: A narrative perspective'. In D. Denborough (ed.), *Trauma: Narrative Responses to Traumatic Experience* (pp. 25–85). Adelaide: Dulwich Centre Publications.

White, M. (2007). *Maps of Narrative Practice*. New York: W. W. Norton & Co.

White, M. and Epston, D. (1990). *Narrative Means to Therapeutic Ends*. New York: Norton.

Winslade, J. (2005). 'Utilising discursive positioning in counselling'. *British Journal of Guidance and Counselling* 33, 351–364.

Winslade, J. M., Crocket, K., and Monk, G. (1997). 'The therapeutic relationship'. In D. Epston (ed.), *Narrative Therapy in Practice: The Archeology of Hope* (pp. 53–81). San Francisco: Jossey-Bass Publishers.

Winslade, J. and Hedtke, L. (2008). 'Michael White: Fragments of an event'. *The International Journal of Narrative Therapy and Community Work* 2, 5–11.

Wolin, R. (2006). 'Foucault the Neohumanist?'. *Chronicle of Higher Education*, 1 September 2006.

Worsley, R. (2008). 'The ground of our relating: Martin Buber's I and Thou'. In S. Haugh and S. Paul (eds), *The Therapeutic Relationship: Perspectives and Themes* (pp. 181–191). Ross-on-Wye: PCCS Books.

Young, J., Saunders, F., Prentice, G., Macri-Riseley, D., Fitch, R., and Pati-Tasca, C. (1997). 'Three journeys toward the reflecting team'. *Australian and New Zealand Journal of Family Therapy* 18, 27–37.

Zimmerman, J. L. and Dickerson, V. C. (1996). *If Problems Talked: Narrative Therapy in Action*. New York: Guilford.

Zimring, F. (2000). 'Person-centred therapy'. In F. Dumont and R. Corsini (eds), *Six Therapists and One Client* (pp. 223–268). London: Free Association Books.

Živković, A. and Hogan, J. (2008). 'Virtual revolution? Information communication technologies, networks and social transformation'. In J. Foran, D. S. Lane and A. Živković (eds), *Revolution in the Making of the Modern World: Social Identities, Globalization, and Modernity* (pp. 182–198). New York, NY: Routledge.

Žižek, S. (2000). *The Ticklish Subject: The Absent Centre of Political Ontology*. London: Verso.

Index

Printed and bound by CPI Group (UK) Ltd, Croydon, CR0 4YY